About the author

One of three girls in an ordinary happy family, Patricia Byrivers developed rheumatoid arthritis while still at school. There was no family history of the disease. She was forced to sacrifice hopes of college and a teaching career for occasional secretarial work when her fingers would allow her to type. Although her joints still bear old scars and she is still dependent on smaller doses of the drugs she has taken for over thirty years, the author is now totally free of pain and can enjoy her great passion in life — boating.

Also published by Century Arrow:

Curing PMT the Drug Free Way *Moira Carpenter*
How to Beat Fatigue *Louis Proto*
The Bristol Diet *Dr Alec Forbes*
A Gentle Way with Cancer *Brenda Kidman*
The Long-Life Heart *Dr Arabella Melville and Colin Johnson*
Overcoming the Menopause Naturally *Dr Caroline M. Shreeve*

GOODBYE TO ARTHRITIS

How to Recognise and Overcome Allergic Arthritis

Patricia Byrivers

CENTURY ARROW

LONDON MELBOURNE AUCKLAND JOHANNESBURG

A Century Arrow Book
Published by Arrow Books Limited
62-65 Chandos Place, London WC2N 4NW

An imprint of Century Hutchinson Ltd

London Melbourne Sydney Auckland
Johannesburg and agencies throughout
the world

First published in Great Britain in 1985
by Century Hutchinson Ltd
First published Century Arrow edition 1986
Reprinted 1986

Royalties from this book are donated to the Help Yourself to Less Pain Society, a self-help group for those who wish to trace the allergic connection to their arthritis.

British Library Cataloguing in Publication Data

Byrivers, Patricia
Goodbye to arthritis: how to recognise
and overcome allergic arthritis
1. Arthritis — Diet therapy
I. Title
616.7'20654 RC933

ISBN 0 09 946730 5

Printed and bound in Great Britain by
The Guernsey Press Co. Ltd
Guernsey, Channel Islands

This book is dedicated to all those who know
the pain of arthritis

Acknowledgements

My sincere thanks to the many people who have helped, eased and encouraged me: my long-suffering parents, dedicated specialists, doctors, hospital staff, family and friends.

Contents

Foreword

By virtue of their position in society, doctors are expected to treat ill-health and disease. To do this they need to make a diagnosis, which is followed either by an operation or more likely the prescription of a drug of sorts. The wide variety of drugs currently used by doctors has only been in existence for two or three decades, but for some unknown reason doctors can't seem to do without them.

Despite the explosion of 'wonder drugs', people in so-called civilised countries seem to be suffering from diseases that were uncommon or frankly rare in the last century and earlier. Humans are developing illnesses that can be called 'chronic degenerative diseases', such as heart attacks, strokes, multiple sclerosis, diabetes and arthritis.

When treating these diseases with drugs, doctors don't seem to realise it is like 'closing the stable door after the horse has bolted'. Doctors rarely actually ask the question 'why?' often enough. Why are these drugs not actually making much difference? Could it be the medical profession is approaching disease from the wrong direction?

To suffer from a crippling disease is bad enough, but to find that the medicines given you don't seem to be working and that no doctor has the answer must be a devastating experience. All the more credit to someone who decides to 'do something for herself'. Even more credit, when she discovers that, despite not being a qualified doctor, she can actually make herself better. I suppose the annoying part is 'if only I had tried this years ago!'

Diseases are given names by doctors which conjure up a picture of the patient. Arthritis is divided into rheumatoid, osteo, gouty, psoriatic, juvenile (Still's disease), and a few other rare types. Patricia Byrivers has introduced a new name – 'allergic arthritis' – into medical terminology. It may yet be found to be more important than all the other types put together.

In describing her experiences and her own method of finding out which foods had a bad effect upon her arthritis and possibly caused it in the first place, Patricia Byrivers must have worked very hard on herself, and must often have wanted to throw in the towel. Having felt well just once, however, after going on to only a few foods for a period of time, she had proof that, if she persevered, she would be able to work it all out in the long run.

What Patricia Byrivers has done by this experience is to discover for herself that arthritis, like so many of today's chronic degenerative diseases, has an underlying cause in the food we all eat. Some people also react badly to chemicals in the environment, such as lead from car and diesel fumes, North Sea gas, perfumes and any one of a number of chemicals so many people use and take for granted today. For the susceptible individual they can spell disaster.

It is a tragedy that no one helped Patricia Byrivers with her food allergies, and equally sad that her experiences have not been taken up actively by her medical attendants to apply to other arthritics. She would certainly have benefited further from dietary supplements early on in the form of vitamins and minerals, but who would have advised her? 'If you are on an average diet,' most doctors would probably have told her, 'you should be getting all the vitamins and minerals you need'. The average diet is what the average person is eating and, quite frankly, the average person is eating a rubbish diet!

There is an obvious need for people who have had experiences of this sort to write about them so that we may all learn. Certainly there are some doctors in Great Britain, albeit still far too few, who are beginning to practise this sort of medicine, and two societies have been formed for medical men, namely the British Society for Clinical Ecology and the British Society for Nutritional Medicine, although the latter welcomes certain non-medical people as Associate Members.

It is my sincere hope that books such as Patricia Byrivers' *Goodbye to Arthritis* will one day become works of historical interest, reminding physicians of the day about the pioneering work of a handful of people. It is at least unlikely that Patricia Byrivers will be ridiculed for what she is saying; not so the poor pioneers of the past like Hahnemann, the originator of homoeopathy, Freud (yes, Freud!), and Pasteur who was laughed at when he asked surgeons to wash their hands before operating!

Whatever method you choose it is best not to stay on a narrow diet for too long without seeking professional advice, or you may become nutritionally deficient. If something works, fine; if it doesn't, don't persevere with it too long. Always try to make sure your diet is nutritionally adequate. Whilst this book has been written by someone suffering from arthritis, it could just as easily have been written by a sufferer from migraine or someone with eczema, asthma, or a set of symptoms that refuses to be neatly categorised. If you can't get anywhere with your current treatment and everyone seems to have given up on you, you may find your symptoms respond to an approach as described in this book.

Dr Patrick Kingsley MB BS FSCE
Treasurer of the British Society for Nutritional Medicine

– 1 –

How Things Used To Be

Many years ago a young woman was sitting on a bus travelling to work, but wishing the bus would crash so she could die. She had neither the energy nor the will to do anything about killing herself, but all her enthusiasm for life had gone.

She had been brought to this low point at the age of just 19 by the constant pain and sheer frustration of rheumatoid arthritis. After several years of the best treatment available by kind and conscientious specialists and general practitioners, together with hospitalisation and strong drugs, she had been told she could not expect any more improvement. There was nothing else to be done but to remain as active as possible for as long as possible, and to continue to take all the prescribed pills. Yet, because she could still just get about, the medics looked upon her as one of their more successfully treated cases!

That morning she had been awakened as usual at 6.30 am by her mother with tea, painkillers and the infra-red lamp set up to try to ease the morning stiffness from her joints. Then she washed and dressed with difficulty, breakfasted, and left the house in time to walk to the bus stop. She walked slowly so as not to display any sign of a limp, for she still had some pride.

On her way to work that morning she was stopped by the District Nurse who happened to be visiting a neighbour.

'Are you all right, love?' she enquired. She had noticed the dreadful bruises on the girl's shins through her tights, and naturally wondered if she was being ill-treated.

'No, no, I'm quite OK' was the embarrassed reply. 'It's the steroid drugs I take – the smallest touch against any furniture, and I have another big, black bruise.'

The delay meant the bus was now in sight, but she was not near enough to the stopping place. She limped along as fast as she could and fortunately her friends saw her predicament and held up the kindly bus driver until she could get there. Their chatter and joking sustained her until she changed to the long-distance bus where she sat alone. Her back ached and did not fit the seat. Her knees hurt to bend up in the narrow space. Above all, her shoulders and hands were in torment as the result of the typing at work – work which she knew she was lucky to get as she was not fully able-bodied. She felt tired and dizzy most of the time and could not see how she could face the future if this was how it was going to be.

Of course, the bus did not crash. She had to get off and walk up the hill to the office, pretend all was well to colleagues and get down to some more of the dreaded typing, which was almost too painful to bear. 'Never mind,' she told herself, 'Saturday tomorrow and a couple of days off.'

'Cheer up, it might never happen.' Her boss had caught her off-guard for a moment and saw a glimpse of the misery behind her usual bland smile.

'There's a telephone call for you,' he said kindly.

Wondering if anything worse could happen, she went to the telephone. It was a young man friend excitedly inviting her to a barn-dance that evening. Assuming she would be delighted to accompany him, he brushed aside all excuses and said he would call for her at 8 pm. Most young women would have been pleased and excited at the prospect, but she simply worried whether she would be able to have a bath and dress in time. This particular friend – horror of horrors – knew little of her illness. So far, she had accompanied him only on jaunts to the cinema and other excursions not calling for much physical activity on her part. She would have to admit that a few steps at a slow dance pace were all she could manage.

Somehow she stumbled through the evening, the events of the day having loosened her joints just enough. To her surprise she even enjoyed herself. At 1 am she crept upstairs to bed.

'Are you all right?' her anxious father called out.

'Yes Dad, I'm fine, thanks, but I'll sleep in in the morning. Good night.'

About ten o'clock the next morning she was awakened by the arrival of her friends of the night before, all ready to go for a swim in the sea at the bottom of the road.

Of course, she had completely stiffened up as a result of her exertions the previous night. 'Tell them I'll follow them in a minute,' she frantically asked her mother, who had relayed the invitation whilst passing pills and drink with one hand and switching on the heat-ray lamp with the other.

She could not manage to walk down the road to join the others that day and many another outing had to be declined on one pretext or another. Because she could just get about, trying desperately hard to look and act normally, she would not admit to being ill if she could avoid it. Perhaps this was a mistake, but if people were sympathetic, her tears, which were always near the surface, would force their way through. Her pretence was a form of self-defence.

A similar pattern of pain and frustration went on for many years. Sometimes the pain was less, sometimes it was more, but all the time her joints were becoming more damaged and it was increasingly difficult to cope.

Looking back now I find it difficult to believe that poor creature was me! For eventually I found a chink of light at the end of the tunnel. I managed to escape from that life sentence of almost constant pain and depression and although I can never be fit enough again to take a proper job or dance, or do many of the things I would like to, some days I have virtually no pain and I am so happy it is like being at a party most of the time – even when scrubbing the floor or cleaning the oven, both of which I can now reach.

This breakthrough came in about 1976 when I eventually

discovered I was allergic to various of the foods I was eating every day (and, incidentally, thoroughly enjoying). After a lot more research I came to the conclusion there must be thousands of people in pain who could help themselves to alleviate it just as I had done, if only they knew how. I am not making any claims for a wonder-cure. I still have rheumatoid arthritis but I and many others have found profound relief from the pain, stiffness and incapacity which are the main symptoms of the disease.

This was the reason I felt I must write this unusually optimistic book about arthritis. After twenty years of increasing pain and decreasing mobility, my prayers to feel even just a little better were answered. These days I feel so well and happy that if I have the odd ache or pain and start to grumble, I firmly remind myself how lucky I am to be able to do so many things I wish to and rush around as much as I do. I quite happily tolerate a restricted diet because it means I no longer have intense pain.

In fact, I have to remind myself just how bad the pain was because it is only natural to forget unpleasant experiences as quickly as possible – a sort of healing amnesia that helps to take away the bitterness of twenty wasted and painful years. One of the worst aspects of rheumatoid arthritis is the realisation that your doctors can do so very little for you. They can offer painkillers and anti-inflammatory drugs, physiotherapy, injections, and eventually operations, but the disease has to take its long, long course. I was given rays of hope from time to time along the lines of 'It might eventually burn itself out', or 'It works in seven year cycles'. All too often it goes on indefinitely.

Resorting to the relevant library, I was confronted with books which described ways of splinting deformed limbs, sleeping in this posture or that to keep limbs relatively straight, exercising regularly and above all keeping the patient cheerful? 'Cheerful about what?' I wanted to know. In the face of all this, because I am so grateful for my recovery after being told by everybody to expect the worst, I made up my mind to tell as many fellow-sufferers as possible. If only a few per hundred try out these safe ideas and obtain some relief without recourse to the drugs which are the usual treatment, then I shall feel I have done just a little to repay the debt I owe to good fortune.

Throughout these twenty-plus years I had short periods of feeling a little better but each remission always ended with a renewal of the pain, weakness and incapacity I knew only too well. Each time there was a further loss of movement in such little things as reaching certain high shelves, fastening clothes, or unscrewing jars. Before my life had really begun, it was gradually slipping out of my grasp, along with too much of the crockery. My world was becoming more and more limited by my physical inability to do things, coupled with my exhaustion from being forced to tolerate too much pain.

At that time I had no possible way of knowing that arthritis could be an allergic condition, nor that I could conduct simple tests at home to ascertain quickly which substances were aggravating my pain. I was simply so desperate for any relief at all that I tried one so-called 'cure' after another. Then, by luck, when these had all failed, I turned to examining my diet. Tracing the foods you are allergic to can be an exciting detective story and very slowly I gradually removed all the items which had been worsening my aches and pains.

The results were worth all the effort. Most of the pain simply went away, while I went on a 'high' of elation which has never completely disappeared, even when I do still have the odd bad day. The difference is that I can usually explain why I am experiencing a little pain and fatigue again, and it is usually because I have not been able to resist eating something which I know I should not. It is as simple as that – cause and effect. I am not a paragon of virtue who eats only raw greens and bean sprouts. My diet is still extremely varied, perhaps more so than before I took an interest in the effects of food on health, because now I think about what I eat and make an effort to extend the range of things I can tolerate.

Nor am I suggesting that following one's own carefully

selected diet is an absolute 'cure' for arthritis. What I am saying is that often it may be perfectly possible safely to alleviate much of the pain, arrest the deterioration of joints and rebuild some of the muscle power which this disease typically causes to waste away. But people like myself still have the disease and some still have to take a lesser amount of the drugs to suppress the symptoms. We certainly continue to need the help and support of doctors, rheumatologists and hospitals. In present day parlance the methods of dietary control described in this book can best be termed 'complementary medicine': a very effective, natural way of losing much of the pain, which is one of the worst aspects of this disease.

I am not suggesting that everyone who has rheumatoid arthritis has an allergy to, say, cheese – far from it. I am afraid there is much more to it than that. But it is clear that many people with arthritis are allergic to certain foods, and can help themselves feel much better than they could ever imagine by carefully investigating which foods are causing the trouble and then eliminating them from their diet.

Once I got over the initial excitement of feeling so very much better that I could stop taking painkillers altogether and reduce my remaining drugs, I realised how important my discovery could be for many others with arthritis. I started to talk and correspond with many people in order to spread the information and by searching I contacted a small society who were campaigning for better recognition and treatment for allergic people in general.

Thinking my discovery would be of value to them I explained it all in a letter to their doctor. I received a very kind reply with some help for my residual problems, but in effect it advised that it was already known in certain medical circles that arthritis could be helped in this way. It had been known about and published in the strictly medical press since the 1930s!

I was very angry. Furious, in fact, to think how I and thousands like me had suffered all those years of pain and increasing disability when the answer was there all the time.

Why had no one told us that we could be making matters so much worse simply by the foods we were eating, even if we did appear to be eating a well-balanced diet? I could not believe such a momentous discovery could lie around on bookshelves and rarely reach the people it ought to be helping.

Many years later, still feeling extremely well and having corresponded with many other sufferers, I have begun to appreciate some of the obstacles in getting it accepted by the public, let alone the medical profession, that certain major debilitating diseases are caused by allergic reactions to certain foods or chemicals.

But as this form of self-help is demonstrably safe and as I feel certain that many people who are in pain at this very moment can be helped, I have set out the whole scenario for you in a non-medical form, so you can try it for yourself or for your child, relative or friend. Ordinary people simply do not read books by doctors for doctors and would not understand their technical language. To put it simply: eating something to which we are allergic day after day aggravates the conditions known as arthritis and makes our pain and joint damage worse. Take away the offending food and you take away the cause of the pain. Then, to a very considerable extent, the damage gradually heals.

Doctors researching in allergic responses seem to be concentrating more on producing pills to treat the symptoms than on examining the causes of allergic conditions. A more sensible approach would surely be to remove the *source* of the trouble if, as in my case, this source is in the diet.

Arthritic pain typically takes two distinct layers in the sufferer. First, there is the general feeling of being ill, with a lack of energy, drive and strength and an overall aching, coupled with inflammation and pain around the joints which discourages movement. Later, as specific joints are progressively damaged, comes the more severe pain which physically limits movement. When you eliminate all or at least your main allergens (foods which aggravate your pain) the first layer of your illness will probably evaporate as if it had never existed.

The second, deeper layer of pain, which is caused by pathological changes which have taken place, such as loss of the lubricating surfaces of joints, can take longer – depending on how long you have had the illness and how much damage has been done. But even this responds eventually, provided the correct diet is persevered with.

When you consider that the pain of arthritis was listed in an article in the American magazine, *Time*, as being one of the worst human experiences, and one of the most difficult to treat, it seems a little obvious to suggest that if you remove the cause the pain will diminish and eventually go, even in long-term cases. But for many people it does.

I am not an isolated case of a patient responding well to this method. There are many more who have tried it and found enormous benefit. I think the reason it has not been more widely recognised is because it is of no advantage just to tinker about with one's diet trying this or that fad in a speculative fashion. After much experimentation and research, and correspondence with other patients, I have been able to compile a list of all the main foods which have increased arthritic symptoms. By going on a trial period of eating none of these foods, you will be able to take advantage of this prior experience and, I hope, find your main allergens straight away. You will then be able to check, by 'challenge testing' each major food group, exactly which foods you really are allergic to, and which ones you can joyfully return to eating.

– 2 –

Early Days

Let me start at the beginning and describe briefly how arthritis crept up on me. That way, similar young sufferers will be able to recognise the early signs themselves.

I was fortunate to start life in an ordinary family with two sisters and parents who loved us and cared for us very well under the difficult circumstances of the Second World War, with all its attendant separations, rationing and air raids. Given the same home background, I have often pondered the mystery of our resulting lives. Sisters numbers one and three are both fit and healthy, whilst I, the middle one, developed rheumatoid arthritis. There is no history of the disease on either side of our parents' families – it just struck out of the blue.

The first sign that I can remember of anything being wrong was a quite excruciating pain in my shoulders. The exact time scale I have forgotten, but I was in my teens and leading an active life when the next symptom developed: a hard swelling between the knuckles of one hand. It was a little sore and showed up when gripping the handlebar of my bicycle. The family thought I had put a bone out of place. Eventually I was persuaded to go to our family doctor. I shall never forget his concerned face as he explained that this was a serious condition for one so young and told me I would have to go to see a specialist at the hospital.

'It was some years before the realisation finally came home to me that, unlike measles and other childhood illnesses, my arthritis was not going to go away.

As in women's clothing, fashions change in the treatment of our various ills and at that time tonsils were medically considered to be the harbingers of germs and the cause of many of our ills. I was despatched to the Ear, Nose and Throat Department where a bemused surgeon asked 'Do you get a sore throat in the area of your tonsils?'

'Well, if you point out where my tonsils are, I can tell you if the rare, slight irritation I experience is in that area' was my equally puzzled reply.

He was surprised and amused to find such ignorance and lack of self-diagnosis in one of his victims, but that did not prevent the removal of my innocent tonsils.

It goes without saying that this treatment did nothing for my arthritis. And as I had never suffered from tonsillitis it hardly cured that. I am just extremely grateful that the fashion at that time happened to be removing tonsils: had I been born a generation earlier, I might well have had my (perfectly healthy) teeth taken out in the same vain hope of finding a cure for arthritis.

I respect the advances made by modern medicine but I do think that over-specialisation has produced a race of specialists with few doctors having the time or inclination to stand back and view an overall picture of cause and effect. If we could encourage some of this great pool of skill and knowledge to be concentrated into maintaining positive health in the first place rather than always relying on our doctors to pick up the pieces after illness has struck, great benefits could be enjoyed by the whole population. Perhaps it is still too early days?

At that time I was feeling too ill and devastated to think clearly, a pity because it is at such crisis points that we require all our faculties. I lived from day to day, struggling to maintain some sort of normal existence whilst drowning in a swamp of pain and disability which I could not understand. My parents, I now realise, had the even more difficult task of caring for me and watching me deteriorate without knowing what on earth to do for the best.

From never knowing what boredom was, my mother and I were reduced to watching afternoon television to help pass the heavy hours, even having little bets between ourselves on the horse-racing. Quite a contrast with the goals of 'A' levels, college and active career which had been projected for me earlier.

At that time I was entering the acute stage of the disease with joints swollen and painful, muscles wasting away visibly and a general ill or 'fluey' feeling. I was entirely wretched most of the time. I did not even reflect on lost opportunities; I was simply feeling too ill. I can remember sitting in a big armchair on my own, facing the cheerful fire with a clock on the mantelpiece and literally wishing the hours away, unable even to hold a magazine up to read – let alone a book from the library. At times like that I could feel my heart racing and pounding in time to the visible movement of the tied sash of my cotton housecoat. Nowadays I realise these were severe palpitations and had I only the knowledge I now have, I could have used these uncomfortable symptoms to assist in diagnosing the wrong foods I was eating and circumventing the only too usual course of rheumatoid arthritis. (See Chapter 9 for the 'pulse test' and other 'challenge tests'.)

Life came down to a miserable existence of lying in bed until lunchtime, then being assisted to wash and dress and come downstairs in great pain, although I was taking many aspirins daily. I ate lunch with difficulty as my shoulders, elbows, wrists and hands were all badly affected, not to mention the pain and stiffness in my jaw which made even chewing unbearable. My mother would give me a light diet of easily managed foods, such as fish, eggs and cheese – rather prophetic as it turned out. And so I would sit, lie down and eat. They were the only activities left.

The monotony was broken twice a week by visits to the out-patients' department at the local hospital where I would have a little physiotherapy aimed at keeping as much movement as possible, with wax baths for hands and feet. It was clutching at straws, for although it was soothing, even in my bemused state I knew it was doing nothing at all to stop the ravages of the disease.

On one of these outings I overheard someone refer to me as 'that poor young crippled girl'. I was devastated. Until that moment I had thought of myself as an ordinary girl who just happened to be ill at the time. More than anything else, this brought home to me the seriousness of my situation. I looked at the other pitiable patients in the clinic, whose ages and disabilities clearly demonstrated the dismal prospects which lay before me. Remarkably, they seemed a comparatively cheerful bunch on the whole, and they hardly ever complained about their sad lot. They appeared in some unknown way to have come to accept they would not get better – indeed would progressively get worse – but they also seemed to accept they could cope with this with help from the specialists and physiotherapists.

I never did become resigned to my fate and from that time on I made up my mind that, come what may, I would live my life as fully as possible. I would also do all I could to improve my health and capabilities, even if this meant feeling a little better in the short-term and perhaps dying young. Quality of life, or at least a little less pain, seemed a worthwhile objective.

To add to my frustrations at that very bad time, I am strictly an outdoor type of person and not very much interested in indoor pursuits such as playing cards, or doing jigsaw puzzles. When I was a child we lived in a modern housing suburb, all laid out in geometrical squares. I would walk to school along plumb straight roads, albeit with some grass and trimmed shrubbery at their edges. I do not know now where I got the mental picture or the idea, but as far back as I can recall I knew I wanted to live in the countryside where there were no uniformly straight roads, nor other houses. From the top of a nearby railway bridge, by standing on tiptoe, I could see distant trees which were all apparently higgledy-piggledy and not at all like the local park where we were sometimes taken to play. At last the day came when I was old enough to follow the path by the railway lines and walk amongst these huge trees. It did not seem to matter too much that it turned out to be the surrounds of a well-manicured golf course! There was a winding footpath with a natural brook in which we caught tadpoles, and many happy hours were spent getting in the way of golfers and enjoying a slightly wilder environment and wider horizon than was possible near my built-up home area.

To this day there is nothing I like better than walking in the utter quiet of a densely wooded area, preferably under the cathedral-like dome of tall ancient trees with no trodden paths and no evidence of any other humans having passed that way; the glimpse of a squirrel racing around and upwards, the distant sighing of the wind in the topmost branches with the only other sound that of a bird warning his mate of my quiet approach.

As I have said, my early childhood was unremarkable. We were an average family with nothing to differentiate us from millions of others. The Second World War obviously caused the adults much worry, but to little girls with no experience of any other way of life, the background of grave news, comings and goings, several billeted 'uncles' and sleeping under a steel Anderson shelter, was all taken as the usual way of living – quite amusing diversions to look forward to!

With the benefit of hindsight we have since learned that the meagre rations which the shortages of war forced upon us were, in fact, good for our health as it was impossible for ordinary folk to over-indulge themselves in any respect. In spite of the very real stress of fear, loss of friends and loved ones, working long hours for little reward and so on, the so-called stress-induced illnesses of heart attacks and ulcers were less evident. They reared their ugly heads during the prosperous period of the 1950s and 1960s, reaching epidemic proportions in Western society of the present day.

During the war years the government still managed to provide extra milk, orange juice, rosehip syrup and cereal food for children, so we were not under-nourished. I remember rejecting my slice of the Sunday joint, for even then meat did not appeal to me. It may not be all coincidence that I am now allergic to milk, wheat and oranges. Apart from the usual infectious illnesses of childhood we were apparently quite fit and walked 1½ miles to school and back twice a day, for school dinners were not so commonly taken in those days. We were rather skinny and our family doctor took pains to reassure our mother that this was our natural build and we would fill out as we grew up.

From what I can remember and have since heard, I must have been a most unrewarding child to bring up, for I was desperately shy and would do all I could to avoid speaking to adults other than those I knew well. Harmlessly, perhaps with good intentions, one particular adopted 'uncle' had not the sense to leave me alone and would pursue me wherever I hid from him. I was literally terrified of him. I was also frightened of the dark, teachers, animals, travelling – almost anything you care to mention. Gradually I overcame most of the outward manifestations of these fears, but it was not until many years later when I discovered and eliminated my allergens that I became fully confident outside the family circle and could speak in company or go out alone at night without suffering the unreasoned terrors of my youth. I still prefer the peace and quiet of our country life, but now feel capable of taking the London Underground, travelling abroad and most situations in my stride. These are just some of the many benefits mentioned earlier.

There is no doubt about it; looking back I was rather a weary child. I always felt tired and in early photos my knees were enlarged. I was so slow that my family nickname was 'Lightning'. But how can a child who has always felt that way know that she is unwell? I presumably accepted a low level of activity and enthusiasm and guessed that was how everyone else felt. Recently an aunt remarked that my lower back was bent from the time I first stood on my feet, but apart from reminding me to hold my bottom in (which I could not do), nobody apparently suspected I was already harbouring the first signs of rheumatoid arthritis.

We were fortunate to live in a seaside town in the south of

England, but were unable to swim in the sea or play on the beach for many years, as it was feared there would be an invasion along the coast. The beaches were mined, and miles of tank-stops and barbed wire prevented us from sampling the full delights of the seaside. Happily, these precautions were never needed as the anticipated invasion never materialised, but we were evacuated from the danger area at one stage to another aunt who lived on the outskirts of London, where of course we were in more danger of being hit by enemy bombers than in our home.

I was later told that the strain of coping with youngsters in the house of a childless, houseproud hostess finally became too much for my mother after my elder sister had proudly written her name on the wallpaper. She decided she would rather take her chances with the invasion forces in her own home! The streets were deserted and I was fascinated to see the grass had grown up between the paving stones in our absence. In due course the scare receded, our neighbours gradually came home too, and life returned to what had become 'normal' for wartime.

Though the streets had been virtually deserted for weeks, there was no sign of any vandalism; no one even thought of boarding up their homes or shops and I do not recall any break-ins. They rightly say that a common adversary and aim gives people a certain camaraderie, together with a will to work together and help each other which was clearly demonstrated during this time. With the benefit of knowledge of later developments in our society and with my much later interest in the effects of the food we eat upon health and behaviour, I cannot help pondering upon such things. For instance there has since been an experiment in an American prison, where inmates had all been admitted for violent crimes. They were put on a diet markedly different from the usual Western fare of cereals, dairy, meat and convenience foods, with plenty of soft drinks and sugary treats.

The behaviour patterns of these prisoners was carefully monitored before and after the change of diet. It was found that because of eating plenty of fresh salads, vegetables and wholewheat bread, not too much meat and virtually no refined sugar or convenience foods, these young men underwent a measurable change to a more reasonable standard of social behaviour.

During the war, this was virtually the diet that was available on rations, as other food, or excess food, was simply not there in the shops. Sweets continued to be rationed for several years after the war was over. The mass preservation of food, together with its adulteration with flavourings and colourings and its preparation into all sorts of tempting, labour-saving instant meals to entice the housewife to part with her money, had not been thought of and were certainly not essential. You were glad to obtain sufficient plain fare to exist on and everyone with the time and a garden supplemented this with as much home-grown produce as possible.

Aside from the occasional air-raid warning and sound of distant explosions, life was uneventful for us children as we continued to attend school and played with friends as children do. We did not have many toys. Those which were around from pre-war days were precious, together with boxes and tins. Even more treasured were the gifts brought home by our father on his rare leave times, which he had made himself in his spare time during his enforced separation.

We children did not really experience fear or feel deprived. To do so, one must understand the reasons to fear and have known a period of plenty in order to compare them. I remember standing at the kerbside in tears one day as a convoy of tanks and lorries rolled past in an endless stream. A kindly passer-by tried to comfort me saying that the war would be over soon, Daddy would be all right, and so on. The real reason for my tears had no such depth. Their origin was very simple. I could not get across the road to school and knew I would be late and in trouble with the teacher. Could it be that we over-emphasise, if not misinterpret, the effects of outside influences on young children? As long as their immediate little world is secure it does not seem necessary to be concerned about them witnessing a bit of reality.

– 3 –

Schooldays

To be perfectly honest, I did not enjoy school much until I went to grammar school. Until that time, most of the educational work I did because I knew I would be in trouble if I did not do it. However, fear of reprisal was a good master because most of the class also passed the dreaded 'eleven plus' examination and moved on to better things. Looking back, it is easy to regret that we were not inspired to learn for the sheer joy of learning, but that was the method of the day. At worst we were all given the basic tools of learning: reading, writing and arithmetic, and we could choose to continue in the quest for knowledge if we wished.

With the more interesting curriculum and more adult attitudes of the next school, my shyness receded somewhat and I began to enjoy learning about the wider world. In fact, I even did well enough to arrange to stay on to the sixth form and choose an academic career. Suddenly, with the arrival of illness, all was put to naught. At first it was a mere inconvenience and made getting to school and the actual work progressively more difficult, and eventually painful and tiring. Walking along the pavements in hard black shiny shoes was agony. It felt as if the whole of the balls of my feet had needles sticking into them with each step. I felt shaky and ill and gradually withdrew from all the physical exercises and games I used to enjoy, such as hockey, netball, tennis and rounders.

Gripping a pen and writing for any length of time caused my

whole arm to ache and the elbow in particular to become permanently painful. The damage is still there and I can feel it at this very moment whilst writing this book. It is not so bad as it was because of the remedial action I took later, which greatly lessened the overall devastating effect of this illness. Treatment at that time was lots of aspirins every day, which had the dual function of easing the pain and bringing down the swelling, but which obviously in no way removed the cause of the trouble.

Next, I went through the pointless tonsil removal episode mentioned earlier. By now, although I was in a lot of pain, my muscles had not wasted away too much and I still led a reasonably active life and to an outsider looked perfectly normal and healthy. That year, during the school holidays, I obtained a temporary job in a famous ice cream parlour, where I would stand at the window and serve soft cornets which I executed beautifully with a flat spoon, after being taught the knack. And if business was slack, as an enticement, I would be delegated to saunter along outside the shop licking an enormous cornet. However, I was grateful for the sit-down when it was my turn to wash up at a little sink under the counter.

I also took great pride in making all sorts of artistically arranged fruit sundaes and knickerbocker glories in tall glass dishes, until we had to limit the number of customers ordering the latter at any one time after I swept too many of the newly washed glasses off the counter by ringing up the cash register at the wrong moment. The drawer leapt out, catching one glass which toppled the rest in a seemingly slow, but unstoppable, domino effect. To their credit, the owners hardly complained as I swept up the pieces. I am delighted to report I recently had lunch in their much expanded business, which is now being run by the younger generation.

That same holiday I also managed to persuade my doctor to sign a medical certificate signifying that I was capable of undertaking a course of boating instruction with the Sea Rangers at Dartmouth. It was wonderful living on a Motor

Torpedo Boat moored in the middle of the estuary, coming and going in small dinghies, having tuition, taking part in competitions and so on. In spite of all my troubles since, there have been very few occasions when I have not been able to indulge my love of the water and sailing. I feel that having an absorbing hobby of this sort has been of tremendous help in persuading me to take calculated chances in extending myself. It would have been all too easy to take the road of least resistance and avoid a lot of pain through unessential exercise.

However, all that was in the future, because my next school year was missed entirely as the rheumatoid arthritis became more severe. I became rapidly worse, with too much pain to move much at all, and was completely dependent upon my poor parents for everything, from feeding, dressing and bathing, to the most important task of company. I did not realise at the time how difficult it must have been for them to cope. None of us had any parallel experience apart from an acquaintance of my grandparents' who came to visit occasionally. She had suffered rheumatoid arthritis from about the age of seventeen and was by then virtually crippled, having led a very deprived and painful life. The poor lady was hardly in a position to paint a very optimistic picture for us.

Most of the time I do not think about my illness at all. I have always, rightly or wrongly, tried to deny its presence in my life. I rarely tell acquaintances that I suffer from it and choose clothes which will hide my damaged shoulders, enlarged knees, curved back and so on. But when I do think about it, I speculate on such things as why it should have happened to me specifically and not to others in my immediate group. If it is allergy based, as I have now proved to my own satisfaction, why was I allergic and not my sisters or classmates? Why does it strike so many women and yet is not purely a women's illness? If it is bound up with the hormonal make-up of women, why is there an infantile form of rheumatoid arthritis which strikes boys and girls alike? I wish I could tell you all the answers, but they are simply not known yet. We do know that many more women than men are affected by other allergic conditions as well as rheumatoid arthritis. New research being conducted right now into hormone treatments for such victims may also throw light on our problems.

It was indeed a hormone that came to my aid when I was eventually admitted to a local general hospital to be confined to bed for an initial three weeks in an ordinary medical ward. At first I was given increased amounts of aspirin, but eventually my digestive system revolted, and instead of dutifully swallowing the tablets as they were dished out, I left them on the locker top until a little mountain accumulated and the staff took the hint that it was no use issuing any more.

One of the alternatives just entering the armoury of rheumatologists at that time was cortisone. Unfortunately, this powerful 'wonder drug' was then very new and, although the kind and conscientious specialist concerned was aware of some of the many side-effects involved, and had hesitated before starting me on these new tablets, there was still much that was not known about it. Nowadays, cortisone and other steroids are seldom given to young or even middle-aged patients as, having once started to take them, it is extremely difficult to stop, and there are many undesirable side-effects. The drug companies are working all the time to find a new substance to alleviate arthritis because so many people suffer from this scourge that the potential market is enormous. Several alternatives are now available for the physician to try in turn until one or other drug or particular combination happens to suit the patient and at least alleviate the worst of the pain.

I strongly advise you to think twice before taking, or being given too many drugs for your illnesses. Do not be afraid to ask your doctor for more information about any prescriptions. Enquire what the action of the drug is supposed to be and what side-effects it has. If he cannot or will not tell you, look it up at your local library. But best of all, try to avoid any long-term pill-taking. See if you can learn from my mistakes and find out whether you can initially control your pain by avoiding eating those foods which are wrong for you.

– 4 –

Allergic Reactions

I wish it were as simple as suggesting that, in order to feel better, all sufferers from rheumatoid arthritis should eat exactly the same diet as I do now. Unfortunately, this is not the case, for every person is different in their chemical reactions and past history; we are each biochemically unique. The offending foods will vary from person to person, but each individual should still be able to trace his own allergic reactions.

One of the chief advantages of this dietary approach to arthritis is that it is utterly harmless. It is quite difficult to achieve and demands a high degree of dedication and even skill, on your part, but it is an approach that cannot possibly make your illness worse, and most people who have tried it seriously have found immense relief. I think one of the reasons the medical profession find it so hard to accept is because there are no nice, neat scientific studies which can be pointed to, nor any one set diet which is always successful. Many people find their General Practitioners or specialists sceptical, if not antagonised, by their request for help in this field. In the face of any disbelief, if not downright disapproval of their self-treatment by diet, sufferers tend to keep quiet about it and continue to treat themselves at home in conjunction with orthodox medical treatment, where they feel they still need it.

How much more satisfactory it would be if their doctor, or a preventative medicine specialist, could help and advise them in their sterling efforts! So approach your medical advisor on the subject – carefully – to gauge his or her reaction. Do not go along, book in hand, to 'tell' him of your 'cure'. If you think it necessary, take his advice in a diplomatic way, so as not to damage your relationship. On the other hand, if he seems sympathetic to your views, count yourself as one of the lucky ones.

Enlightenment is slow to get through, especially to medical schools where, I am reliably informed, instruction on staple food allergy is just about non-existent at the time of writing. Let us hope that with growing pressure from patients who have benefited, this whole subject will become respectable and an accepted part of teaching and treatment, to the great benefit of all.

Until recently, the only types of allergy most people had heard of were such things as hayfever, rashes or other symptoms which came and went and thus could be relatively simply accounted for by allergens such as pollens in the air, shellfish or strawberries. The victims could then avoid eating the offending items or take drugs for their hayfever. It is little wonder there has not been much progress in this field, because each allergic person has his own individual set of symptoms and of foods or other items which trigger them off. Our set of symptoms just happen to have been labelled rheumatoid arthritis, but we could equally well be contending with any one or combination of troubles from migraine, asthma, eczema, indigestion, fatigue, to virtually all the illnesses which are collectively known as the degenerative diseases.

The methods which I am trying to describe to you of eliminating the items which may be causing your aches and pains could possibly be equally effective in treating virtually any of the longterm medical conditions; I just happen to have had rheumatoid arthritis and so have studied this aspect.

More and more it is being realised that human beings are literally made up of what they eat. It is just as important to avoid eating things which disagree with you fundamentally as it is to ensure you consume sufficient proteins, starches, fats, roughage, minerals, vitamins and trace elements to provide the building bricks for nature to fuel and repair your body. Western countries are becoming much more health conscious and we are encouraged to take more exercise, eat less fat, stop smoking and look after ourselves. The advice is rather generalised and comes too little and too late for many.

What has emerged after much trial and error is that many people with the types of degenerative illnesses mentioned above have what is known as a 'staple food allergy'. No one knows why they have such a reaction, but once you realise what is happening it is possible to reverse the reaction and thus mitigate, if not entirely eradicate, the symptoms of your illness. Repeatedly eating or drinking the same type of food or drink every day – in some cases at every meal – can trigger off a kind of revulsion by the body which, in effect, says, 'Enough's enough, I cannot cope with this eating pattern any longer.' The much battered defences finally break down and the reaction becomes an illness.

We should remember that primitive societies, although on a rather restricted diet, dictated by the circumstances of what they can produce locally just to survive, do not exhibit signs of Western diseases. Their food is usually fresh, organically grown, unrefined and does not have the doubtful benefit of the many additives to which we are exposed unless we make a really stupendous effort to avoid them.

The comparison in health between different cultures and lifestyles is a fascinating study. For example, in remote Asian and African areas cooking is all done on wood or dung fires at ground level. Everyone squats on the ground to eat or work because there are very few other seats. Even the venerable elders adopt this attitude with grace and ease, flexing knees and hips like children – no arthritis there. In Britain it is difficult to find a middle-aged, never mind older adult who could perform this feat, even if they do not specifically suffer from any disease. The only ones who can are trained dancers, keep-fit addicts, and those conscious enough of their health to attend yoga classes and so on in their spare time.

There could be several explanations, but no one really seems to know the true answers. It could be simply that, if people are living at ground level all the time, joints are not permitted to stiffen up. Equally, the reason could be that we are simply too fat. Just watch examples of thin and fat people sitting with one leg crossed over the other. The legs of the thin person lie elegantly alongside each other, or even cross twice with the toe tucked behind the ankle. The overweight person's leg, if they manage to hitch it over at all, is held out by the excess tissue. But neither can this be the whole answer, because many arthritics are almost too thin with their wasting muscles and lack of appetite. Similarly, it is not that they do not want to move their joints in order to execute even the tiny chores of everyday living. It is simply that they cannot do so because the damage done by the disease physically prevents movement.

So if it is not just being thin or taking regular exercise, it must be something else. My own first hand experiences of this whole scenario, not to mention the life histories of other sufferers, cause me to remain unshakeably convinced that the secret must be in the food they eat.

An example of a disease caused by harmful eating habits, and a disease which has become such a scourge that even the Government has been forced to make recommendations on better diets, is the alarming incidence of high blood pressure and heart disease. Slowly it is being recognised that many deaths by heart disease could probably have been avoided if the victims had been advised not to eat dairy foods, eggs and animal fats in excess. What usually happens is that, if the first heart attack is not fatal, the patient is put on a strict diet to reduce his weight, thus taking a little of the stress off the damaged heart, and reducing his intake of the cholesterol which sticks to the walls of arteries, gradually clogging them up. This cholesterol accumulation starts early on and builds up until disaster strikes. Post mortem examinations of the heart and arteries of some young accident victims show signs of this lethal build-up from their teens. Early changes are visible even in eight to ten year olds. How much more sensible it would be if parents were advised *not* to give their families plenty of milk, cream, eggs, cheese and fatty meat, suet and fried food, in the first place, and told to replace these foods with more fresh fruit and vegetables. An argument often put forward as an obstacle to this type of diet is the high cost of fresh fruit and vegetables, particularly in winter. However, if this is offset against the large savings which can be made on the milkman and butcher's bills, an overall credit balance is usually effected.

– 5 –

The Addictive Nature Of Allergies

One of the most difficult things about food allergy is that the victims usually do not recognise the cause of their illness. In fact they tend to thoroughly enjoy their food, and cooking and dining often play a large part in their lives. This is because the foods which are causing the trouble frequently turn out to be the very ones they are eating at almost every meal and which they feel they cannot possibly manage without. Just like heavy drinkers or smokers, people who have a staple food allergy have become dependent, or hooked, on particular foods and their reactions work in a similar fashion.

Before the smoker took his first puff of nicotine, he (or she) was perfectly healthy and able to cope with life's ups and downs without the support of a temporary 'lift' from a cigarette. For a while they would be able to continue to smoke or not, but once the duration and frequency of the dose reached a certain level, dependence would be inevitable and the only way to get back to that happy state of coping with their minor urges or problems, or even simply to feel all right, would be to light up another cigarette. The same story applies to the drinking of alcohol. At an infrequent social level it is acceptable, but if the habit becomes too regular and intake too high, problems arise. The body has become addicted to a daily dose and there are real problems if the supply is withdrawn. It can be done, but as any reformed heavy smoker or ex-alcoholic will tell you, it is only achieved by understanding the problem and exerting sufficient willpower to survive those first testing days of withdrawal.

In a similar way to tobacco or alcohol, staple food allergy constantly makes the sufferer feel bad, maybe manifesting itself as a headache or, in the case of rheumatoid arthritis, continuous joint pain and connected troubles, sometimes less, sometimes more, but always present.

Let us take as an example one prevalent cause of pain in rheumatoid arthritis: gluten. Gluten is the sticky substance present in wheat and other flours which makes it possible to knead and stretch dough. It is also present in several other related grains such as oats and barley. We all consume large quantities of gluten, starting perhaps with a breakfast of porridge, or muesli with toast to follow. Then we might have a mid-morning bun or biscuit, followed by a cooked lunch, often accompanied by a bread roll, and with soups, gravies and sauces all thickened with the gluten contained in the flour. Gluten is also in the pie crust around the meat and usually in the pudding which follows. Afternoon or high tea is traditionally a time for more bread, biscuits and cakes, whilst the evening nightcap is a natural time to have a biscuit. With such an all-pervasive food component, it is not surprising some sensitive people become allergic to gluten as their system literally rebels against the constant barrage it is asked to cope with.

Yet, at the same time, the susceptible person may be apparently thoroughly enjoying his or her food because no direct connection can be felt between the food and the pain. In fact, what happens is, if the victim goes for long without the guilty food, he or she begins to feel a need for it as a 'pick-me-up'. Just as the smoker reaches automatically for a cigarette, the allergic person will choose a meal with plenty of his particular allergen in it. For a short time this will indeed make them feel a little better, until the effect wears off, when they will begin to feel the need for the next jolt of gluten. It may sound all very unlikely, but I know from my own experience that this is only too true. It is most improbable that the victim will equate the yearning for a certain food with feeling better; he will simply feel he likes or fancies this particular food rather than another – it is more satisfying. Clinically, this effect is called 'masking'.

This situation can, and has, gone on throughout whole lifetimes without ever being detected. It is not so easy as just stopping eating whatever the substance is which is making you feel ill. In the first place, how do you know which item it is? It could be coffee, or eggs, meat, peanuts, or a particular fruit or vegetable, tea, sugar, milk or even additives or colourings. All these and many more substances in some foods have been implicated in different people's illnesses.

But do not despair, there are ways of eliminating this array of potential criminals.

One of the quickest and simplest tests is to ask yourself which food out of all you eat is your favourite – not a special now-and-again treat but the food (or drink) which you take most frequently and feel you really cannot do without. This is the one likely to be the culprit. Let us suppose you drink ten cups of strong coffee (or tea) daily and feel this might be a good place to start. To break this down, the next question to ask is whether it is the tea (or coffee), the milk or the sugar which is the ingredient harming you, whilst at the same time giving you a temporary lift.

Full of enthusiasm and hope you decide to forsake coffee or tea for a few days and drink something else. Do not change over to all milk or to dubious highly coloured drinks. Try to stick to water with a pure fruit juice now and again as a treat, or you could spoil the results of your experiment. Do not expect to feel better at once. Just like the heavy smoker or alcoholic you are treating a suspected addiction *and must expect withdrawal symptoms.* For a few days you may feel worse rather than better and you will be tempted time and again to have just one cup. If this happens to you, take heart, for it is a sure sign you are on the right track and will soon begin to feel better without your dependence on a roasted bean or the dye and tannin soaked out of a dried leaf with the aid of boiling water.

Once you get through the first few days you should begin to feel better and better, but there is still the temptation of a relapse to former habits. The longing to taste your one-time favourite food or drink lingers for some considerable time.

I did not have the benefit of this trick, or even of knowing that all my troubles were quite probably allergy based. As a result I had fallen into what now seem with the benefit of hindsight to be some very poor eating habits. During the war, the Government, aware of the shortage of sufficient proper food, issued extra milk, orange juice and Ministry of Food cereal for babies and young children. Many of the foods we now treat as commonplace were unobtainable due to the blockading of shipping to try to starve our islands into surrender. Consequently I can clearly remember my first orange, banana and pineapple. As a growing child I had an intermittent watery, itchy rash on my hands and between the fingers. It was treated with creams and lotions, together with admonishments not to scratch, for many years before I realised it was simply caused by the zest spraying out of the skin of oranges when I peeled them. I continued to consume the fruit with gusto if an immune person could be persuaded to peel it for me, and never had any more rashes as a result. Could it be, I wondered as I slowly unravelled the cause of my allergies years afterwards, that I had experienced an overdose of orange juice as a child as a result of the Government's commendable efforts to keep babies topped up with vitamin C? The family doctor was made aware of this discovery about my reaction to orange peel, but with the later onset of rheumatoid arthritis it was never mooted that I might be an allergic type of person.

It was only after years of pain and disability in spite of the very best treatment available, together with an average of a month in hospital every two years for injections in the worst joints, physiotherapy and all sorts of treatment, that I eventually realised I was deteriorating to a point where I simply would not be able to cope in the future. Just to accidentally catch my thumb in my clothing, even quite gently when dressing, would bring tears to my eyes and stop all progress for some minutes until the pain subsided. Brushing and attending to my hair was a task to be put off as long as possible until the worst of the morning stiffness had worn off. Even then it was a painful struggle, pushing my arms up against shoulders and elbows which did not want to bend by the device of resting one elbow on a special little shelf and gradually lowering the rest of my body.

A particularly low point was reached when on coming out of hospital after a month of treatment and a change to a new type of steroids, I felt even worse than when I went in. It was January – the very worst time for arthritics, as the cold emphasises their aches and pains. Like most chronically ill people, I had not the money available for sufficient heating, for while you are ill, there is not much opportunity for making money in this competitive world.

A few days later there was a big winter storm and tidal surge in the North Sea, which continued up the river near where I lived and over the flood bank. The water which escaped over the bank flooded the land on which our house stood. Those people who have experienced salt water flooding will know the full implications of the devastation it causes to carpets, furniture and decorations. The salt remains in the walls and will seep through new decorations for ever unless the plaster is hacked off and the walls re-rendered with concrete. The salt is almost impossible to wash out of carpets and soft furnishings. Ovens, washing machines, sewing machines simply do not work any more and their bases rust away. Treasured trees and garden plants all die.

After a day or two of trying to rescue my belongings and help mop up I felt so ill I could do no more and lay down on a wet settee in the middle of all the chaos and hoped not to wake again.

Now, once again with the benefit of hindsight, I realise that the extra aches and pains were caused not just by the results of the flood, but because, with no electricity and cooking facilities, I was existing on quick snacks of all the very foods to which I was unknowingly allergic.

Out of this dreadful experience came some good. For the first time I actually felt nauseated and began to wonder if I was somehow being poisoned. In a frantic search for relief my over-enthusiastic imagination ran riot to the extent of coming to feel maybe my own disease could have been caught by eating the meat of animals who had somehow contracted it. At the time I knew nothing about allergies and there were never any articles about them in the popular press. I resolved to stop eating any meat just in case it helped. I was on the right track for the wrong reasons and unfortunately, on the best advice I could obtain, I substituted a lot of cheese to provide the protein I was no longer getting from meat.

It was an easy step for me to take as I had never been keen on meat, but had always been prepared to eat cheese at any opportunity. In fact, I recall coming in from school and devouring at least six cheese sandwiches for tea quite regularly.

Had I ever been told about the addiction aspect of allergies I would naturally have suspected cheese to be the culprit first. But in the absence of any information about food allergies it was several more frustrating years before I got around to giving it up. The results were dramatic despite the fact that one doctor had confirmed that cheese would be very good for me. The pain began to recede after only three days, the muddled thinking I had experienced on and off for years disappeared and I went on a 'high' which has lasted for a decade. I was immensely grateful to feel better. The relief was so enormous as to be indescribable. I cannot understand why all those who are in pain are reluctant to try it for themselves. Of course an obvious reason is they have not been told, so in the 1970s I started writing a contribution to the book *Help Yourself to Less Pain*.

One lady who appeared to me to be deteriorating each time I contacted her, and was obviously in considerable pain, told me that eating was the one pleasure she had left in life and she was not prepared to give certain things up even if it meant her health would improve.

I can sympathise with this attitude because I am asking you

to break the habits of a lifetime at a time when you are presumably feeling very low with pain. I do not know how to convince you of the value of experimenting to see if you have a food allergy except to say that although I missed my cheese for a couple of years I have got used to and thoroughly enjoy the substitutes. Today, when preparing cheese dishes for others I am not even tempted to try a little – in fact if I get some on my fingers I hasten to wash it off because its associations with pain are so strong that it now revolts me.

After a while on a cheese-free diet, I went to a party where the charming hostess, a culinary expert, had, out of deference to my diet, provided vegetable soup with cream, trout cooked in butter, homegrown raspberries and fresh cream and delicious coffee with more cream. You have probably guessed the results. By the end of the evening I could only just get out of the armchair and put on my coat to go home. The next day I continued to feel quite dreadful – not sick, you understand – but full of aches and pains, just as quickly as that. Three days later the effects finally wore off and the lesson was well learned. It was not only cheese that was upsetting me but, quite logically, the milk from which it was made, together with butter, cream, yoghurt, dried milk, tinned milk and everything connected with cow's milk, even whey products in tinned goods and margarine.

I felt even better with no milk products, but occasionally experienced a slight increase in pain, about which I would grumble, even though such days would have been termed 'good days' only a short while earlier. In this way I was gradually able to eliminate the rest of the foods which were contributing in a lesser way to my aches and pains. For the first time in twenty years I began to enjoy life. One of my greatest pleasures was to give my long hair a good brush as strength returned to my arms. The movement did not improve initially for the joints had been too damaged, but as the pain receded I could use my limbs more, thus increasing muscle power. Even now, as the years pass I notice slight improvements in movement.

Once established on my new regime and feeling fairly secure, with the approbation of my specialist I began the long and difficult task of reducing my intake of drugs. The moment I started improving I thankfully stopped taking any regular painkillers because they were simply no longer necessary, and I reduced the steroids little by little until I reached a much lower dose.

– 6 –

Discovering Your Food Allergens

Staple food allergies are extremely difficult to track down unless you make a determined effort and have some excellent guidance as to how to go about it. There are many diets recommended for arthritis sufferers, each with its own faithful followers because it worked for *them.*

Of course each one works for some and not for others because, once you realise arthritis has allergic connections, it follows that no two allergic people are quite the same. We are all individuals with considerably different physical make-ups and personal experiences, so our reactions to various foodstuffs definitely vary too.

So let us get it straight right now that there is no one diet to alleviate arthritic pain in all victims. Each person has to arrive at his own solution, his own *individual* diet which will totally exclude the foods to which he is allergic.

It is never too soon and never too late to try this approach. The longer you have had the disease, the more appreciative you will be of any improvement in your health; but if the disease has gone on for many years irreversible changes will have taken place in the tissues involved, so although the pain recedes, the limitations on movement remain, and will only improve slowly. Your general health should improve too – to such an extent that it has been known for old acquaintances not to recognise victims and to find it difficult to believe the change.

I do not suggest you will be entirely 'cured', but like me you will feel more able to cope, be more cheerful and less of a burden on friends and loved ones, not to mention the National Health Service! I still have residual problems and tire quickly – although I try to build up more stamina by extending my activities within reason. It is still frustrating not to be able to keep up with my contemporaries and do as much as I would like, but I remind myself of how I once was and am deeply grateful.

Another difficulty with leaving it so long before discovering the foods which are literally poisoning you to the extent of causing damage to your joints, is that the toxicity builds up and you are able to tolerate a smaller and smaller range of foods as time goes on. Then, if you eventually trace your allergic foods, there tends to be one main one and several subsidiary ones, all contributing in different ways to your problems.

One of the aims of this book is to reach those young people who are attending clinics in those first bewildering years of acute pain and increasing disability. If they are helped to track down the main cause of the trouble early on and the foods that are causing it are avoided for the rest of their lives, they may be able to short-circuit the at present inevitable course of rheumatoid arthritis. Because they will never know the full implications of what they have missed they may not be as delighted as us 'old hands'. But if even one young woman avoids the usual story of ruined lifestyle and constant pain then all my struggles, experiments and effort will have been worthwhile.

Through research and contact with others on diets to relieve arthritis, I have been able to compile a list of foods and drinks which have been found to contribute to this disease in many people. You will see this list is fairly extensive, but it does not mean that everyone with arthritis is allergic to every item on the list, nor that it will be quite safe for you to eat any food which does not appear. This will be explained and discussed as we go along. Do not take fright.

The list published here is intended purely as a guide to

which foods are likely to be implicated and is an advance from starting with no knowledge at all. I have put the worst and most frequent offenders at the top of the list and descend to the ones that only affect a few people, or which affect people to a lesser extent. I am indebted to those who have taken the trouble to write in with their findings and take this opportunity of thanking them here. If you wish to assist others in the future, please let me know the results of your own findings, good or bad (see address of the Help Yourself to Less Pain Society at the back of the book).

Foods and Drinks which are Common Allergens in Cases of Rheumatoid Arthritis

1. *Cow's milk* and all dairy produce, ie fresh, dried, skimmed or tinned milk; cheese of all sorts; butter; cream; yoghurt; whey added to tinned and prepared foods, margarine etc; prepared puddings and ice cream with milk or cream added to them
2. *Wheat grains/gluten*; Anything made with ordinary wheat flour, oats, rye or barley; therefore all ordinary bread, biscuits, pastry and cakes
3. *Wheat bran*
4. *Ordinary thickeners* (which usually contain corn-starch) for soups, gravies, sauces and puddings
5. *Eggs*
6. *Beef* and all products derived from it such as suet, dripping and lard
7. *Lamb*
8. *Pork* including sausages, bacon, ham and luncheon meat
9. *Additives*; Artificial colourings, preservatives, flavourings, and so on

10 *Fruits*; Oranges; lemons; grapefruit; strawberries; raspberries; rhubarb; gooseberries; apples; pineapple; plums; other fruits

11 *Drinks* and preserves made from the above fruits

12 *Corn* and all its derivatives eg cornflour, cornoil, cornflakes

13 *Coffee*

14 *Tea*

15 *Drinking chocolate* and similar hot drinks, most of which contain milk or malt, and some of which contain wheat

16 *Herrings* (rare)

17 *Peanuts*

18 *Other nuts*

19 *Sodium salt*; Sea salt

20 *Alcoholic drinks* if based on any of the above foods to which you are allergic, eg beer, ale and spirits, almost all of which are made from grain

21 *Spices* used in excess

22 *Sugar* where it is made from a particular grain to which you are allergic. Most people with grain allergies are likely to have problems with cane sugar and corn syrup but not with beet sugar

23 *Tomatoes*

24 *Vinegar*

25 *Mushrooms* and other fungi

26 *Yeast*

If after reading this long list of all your favourite foods you are undeterred, we will now discuss ways of applying this knowledge.

By far the quickest, best and most effective way is to eliminate every item on the list for at least two weeks, to see if you improve without them. If you do, and it is the rare person who does not, then simply try adding one of the suspect items at a time, preferably at three-day intervals, to see if your symptoms return. If they do, put that item on your list of foods to avoid. If you experience no adverse reactions, you can joyfully return to eating that food – in moderation, of course.

It all sounds too easy to be true, doesn't it? But there are a few practical difficulties which I will endeavour to help you with.

If you really cannot contemplate such a large upheaval in your lifestyle and eating habits, an alternative would be to try leaving out one item (or a group) at a time. Although this is simpler to cope with at a practical level, it prolongs the time of the experiment and could be unsuccessful because, if (as is highly likely) you are allergic to several of the items, eliminating one guilty food will not bring much benefit while others are still contributing to your aches and pains. The exception would be if you were lucky enough to strike your main irritant right away, when you would feel so much better overall that it should be possible to continue to sort out the lesser ones gradually.

Should you decide to try this Russian roulette approach, I strongly recommend you take first the two offending groups, milk and wheat (and everything that is made from them), closely followed by eggs and red meat.

You may think that if you cannot eat any of the listed foods, even for only two weeks, there will be so little left you will be constantly hungry. I assure you this is not the case. There are many foods left for you to enjoy. By the very nature of the problem, because people tend to become allergic to foods eaten regularly, the ones which are left are the most unusual.

To give you an idea, here is a list of foods which have been found to be fairly safe for most arthritics to use. There can be no guarantees, as you may be unusual and have an allergy to any one of them. They are given basically in a replacement order of the previous list of suspect items.

Foods Relatively Safe for Arthritics to Eat

1 Soya milk; non-milk creamers; sunflower or safflower oil margarine

2 Rice flour; potato flour; soya flour; gluten-free flour if you are allergic just to the gluten and not to the grain as a whole

3 Soya or rice bran

4 Arrowroot or agar agar

5,6,7,8 Fish of all kinds; chicken; turkey; game; legumes such as dried beans, peas and pulses

9 Fresh, unadulterated foods

10 Bananas; peaches; grapes; pears

11,13,14,15 Herb teas; chicory; water, hot or cold

16 All other fish unless you know any in particular which do not suit you

17,18 Most nuts are all right, but test out singly

19 Potassium salt substitute

20 Alcoholic drinks brewed from foods which suit you. Here you will have to do your own detective work to discover basic ingredients. Homemade wines from root vegetables appear to be a good alternative

21 Herbs; freshly ground pepper; mustard; garlic

22 Honey

23 Use beetroot, grated carrot or radishes to add colour to your salad

24 Wine vinegar used very sparingly is usually acceptable; use olive oil on salads

25 Gluten-free baking powder

Throughout this book I have referred to 'testing' the various foods involved. This needs to be done in as objective a way as possible. You will need to keep a notebook or diary of exactly what you ate and drank and how you felt meal by meal and day by day. It is useful to lay this out as in the sample given. The list of symptoms you write in will be your own most troublesome ones, ie 'pain in shoulders'; 'right wrist'; 'left foot'; 'headache'; 'constipation'; and so on. Then, each time you make an entry in your chart, decide on a scale of 0 to 10 (0 being no pain, 10 being the worst you ever experience). This gives you a shorthand way of quickly completing your record. It is all too easy to cheat yourself and feel that the odd bun or ice cream you know you ought not to have had is not worth entering, but please try to be brutally honest and put it all down, or you may never come up with the correct conclusions.

Now that you have your record book prepared and resolve hardened as to what you are going to test, simply exclude that food group or groups from your diet for a fortnight, carefully noting down what you do eat and how you feel. Do not forget that, if for the first few days you feel decidedly off-colour and long to get your teeth into the forbidden items, this probably means you are on the right track because you are suffering the withdrawal symptoms and increased aches and pains discussed earlier. Hold on to your optimism, for it will be difficult to resist taking the easy course. It will need a lot of self-discipline.

Let us assume you are made of strong stuff and successfully survive the first difficult few days and begin to feel better. Congratulations: wonderful, isn't it? While you continue on your rather restricted diet you will continue to improve and allow your body to clear away accumulated poisons.

Now we come to the all-important tests to confirm which of 'The List' are your own personal allergens. Assuming you took

Sample Page of your Food and Reaction Diary

The list can be taped to one side of an ordinary exercise book to save writing it out too often.

Date and time
All food and drinks (no cheating)
Medications
Pulse rate before, immediately after and 20 mins after meals
Visits to the toilet
Mood varying between '0': top of the world and '10': despair
Fatigue not caused by exercise
List of other symptoms that apply specifically to you eg:
Pain in shoulders
Right wrist
Left foot

No 1 first and have had no milk or dairy products for two weeks, at your next meal have a reasonable helping of whatever form you have been missing most. A glass of cold milk, a creamy rice pudding, cauliflower cheese, a plain chunk of cheese, cream trifle – go on, be a devil and enjoy it. But do not change anything else about your diet; only one thing at a time.

In the excitement, do not forget to enter it in your diary along with how you felt just before. Then go about your business and forget about it. The results can vary enormously from nothing, in which case you are fortunate and can continue to enjoy milk and all things connected with it in suitable moderation, to the other end of the scale when almost forgotten aches and pains return with dramatic speed and intensity. I, for instance, know within twenty minutes if I have slipped up and eaten something with milk in a seemingly innocent dish at friends' or in a restaurant. Curry thickened with cream or yoghurt is hard to detect and you cannot always spoil the atmosphere by demanding to know how things have been cooked. But I can tell afterwards by the aches and pains, together with the fluid retention which makes my fingers swell so that rings which slipped off readily before dinner are now held fast on a puffy finger.

If the dose is not repeated, the effects of an attack of this sort generally wear off in the next day or two and can be speeded up by taking a heaped teaspoon of bicarbonate of soda in water to help neutralise the acids which have been formed. The symptoms can be helped by a paracetamol if really necessary, but even these mild painkillers persist a surprisingly long time in the body and can have adverse effects. Keep them for emergency use only, and do not gradually slip into a routine of taking them every day.

In between these two extreme reactions to eating the offending food are many shades of reaction from indigestion, pain in one joint only, general aches, to headaches, return of confusion, irritability, and so on. This denotes a certain amount of allergic reaction which, if you were to continue to eat that particular food, could build up to major troubles again.

After a fairly long period of abstinence it is sometimes possible for the body to rid itself of these milder reactions and be able to tolerate the allergen again in small, occasional quantities. You can readily test this periodically and, if successful, may then permit the use of, say, margarine with whey in it, or enjoy the occasional treat of a bar of chocolate. Should you revert to the constant use of milk in tea, cream on fruit and so on and find your aches gradually returning, then at least you will know the cause and will have to again completely break the habit if you want to regain your freedom from pain.

All that has been said here regarding the testing of milk applies equally to the wheat and grains group, although reactions are usually a little slower to appear.

Here is a case history in her own words of a person with long-term severe rheumatoid arthritis, who was fortunate to discover and eliminate her allergy to gluten. You will note that because of the length of her illness she had multiple allergens and (as is often the case) many different symptoms, all of which were helped.

> At the age of 14 I developed Still's Disease, now called Sero Positive Juvenile Rheumatoid Arthritis, and was very badly crippled within the year. I was allergic to most antibiotics, penicillin and aspirin and I only just recovered from pneumonia and boils caused by a reaction to an antibiotic. I transferred hospitals and was taken off Prednisolone, which had given me relief for a while. At this new hospital it was found I could take Nuseals (Sodium Salycilate), a form of aspirin, and this I was given in large doses until my head rang with buzzing and music! I was still bloated from the effects of the Prednisolone and after nine months I was put on a 1,000 calorie diet. It was from then I started to improve, much to the doctors' surprise and delight.
>
> After 18 months in hospital I was fit enough to start Technical College to finish my education. During this time my regular eating habits during the week were two meals a

day, one at school and a meal with my parents when they had their dinner at night, only eating more bread and cakes at weekends. With 8 Nuseals a day my rheumatoid arthritis was stable, but I suffered from very bad migraines most weekends. These continued throughout my student and working life.

I married in 1968 and had my daughter, Rachel, in 1972. Six months after having my child I had to have a second hiatus hernia operation. During this, complications developed and I was on a sugar drip for two months. During that time all symptoms of my arthritis disappeared, only to return when normal food was eaten again. Nine months later, after my annual check up with my doctor, I was told to feed myself up, and was put on protein tablets. This caused a flare-up, making me nearly as bad as when I first had rheumatoid arthritis. Only the new drug Azathioprine settled my system down so normal life was possible.

In January 1977 my arthritis was stable, with two 125mg Azathioprine, 4 Nuseals and 10 Distalgesic a day, when I decided to make my own bread. Over the next couple of months I started a flare-up for no apparent reason. When a new doctor, standing in for my regular doctor who was in hospital, noticed that my monthly blood tests were showing increased arthritic activity, he was puzzled and came to see me. By this time (March) I could hardly walk and had increased my daily dose of painkillers considerably. During our conversation he was able to tell me exactly when my blood test results had started to deteriorate, which coincided with my making my own bread after Christmas.

He pointed out that with the amount of bread I was eating, what could be doing the damage was the gluten in the flour which was known to cause illness in some people. I agreed to try a gluten-free diet for a week to see if there was any change in my condition. I never saw the new doctor again as he moved to another practice, but the amount of relief I felt in that week was enough to persist with the diet.

The previous year, 1976, I had had an operation to stiffen

a wrist, and the week in bed, coupled with a breakfast each day of bread rolls, had made my knees very painful and swollen. At the time I had put it down to being made to stay in bed for a week. So now in May 1977, when I went into hospital for my left wrist to be done in similar circumstances, I decided to keep to my gluten-free diet. This time my knees were perfect, rested and with all the swelling gone. This convinced me that my diet, although sometimes a nuisance, was worth sticking to, and at my next check-up with my regular doctor I managed to convince her to allow me a prescription for gluten-free flour.

After a year of excluding wheat, rye and barley, I had reduced my Azathioprine to one tablet a day and my Distalgesic to four. During this time I noticed that some Mondays and Tuesdays I was stiff and my ankles were painful. The stiffness coincided with having eaten a joint of beef over the weekend. By gradual deduction over the next year I found that cheese and egg yolks also caused stiffness and so I took them out of my diet too.

Finally, in March 1980, when I went into hospital to have a knee replacement operation, I was taking only one Azathioprine a day. I was given just a gluten-free diet and within two days I was requiring painkillers. When my diet was changed to gluten-free, no beef, eggs and cheese, I was able to make do without painkillers again, but I was drinking more milk than I usually have at home and my stomach started to show coeliac symptoms. I was allowed soya milk and my stomach improved.

I have now become migraine free, only having one last year. I am also completely drug free, having been weaned off the Azathioprine a year ago!

Celia Crouch

– 7 –

Coping With Your New Diet

Once you know the items which have been aggravating your rheumatoid arthritis, you will soon find that some are easier to find substitutes for than others. I have made a few notes which I hope will assist you, and I am always interested in ideas and recipes which can be passed on to make food more interesting on a restricted diet.

I went through three distinct phases on this diet. *Phase I*: excited and happy to be better, experimenting daily and treating the whole thing as an interesting challenge. *Phase II*: bored and slightly envious of others eating anything with impunity; embarrassed when eating out. *Phase III*: entirely used to and happy with the diet. No longer treating eating so much as a social occasion, but still enjoying my food.

Living Without Milk and Milk Products

Milk seems to be used in just about everything we eat, but once you get used to the idea of excluding it you will find it is not as essential as we have been led to believe. Should you establish that you really do have an allergic reaction to cow's milk, it is well worth obtaining some goat's or sheep's milk and testing for these most carefully. You can then continue to eat more or less as before, simply substituting goat's or sheep's milk, cream and cheese in all your usual recipes. These products freeze well and a supply can be kept in the freezer to obviate too many long trips to the nearest supplier.

Sunflower oil margarine

Sunflower oil margarine is an excellent substitute for butter and after a while you will find you prefer the taste of it. Many people find they can tolerate the small amount of whey (a waste milk solid product) in some soft margarines, but there are some completely vegetable oil products available at health food shops. Commercial cakes and biscuits often contain milk, butter or suet, all of which should be avoided.

Non-milk based creamers

Non-milk based creamers in tea or coffee (if you are still using these) are quite an acceptable substitute and very quick and easy to use. It is also convenient to carry a small container of powder in your pocket to have in black tea or coffee when in cafés or visiting acquaintances who have not been forewarned. They can also be used to make sauces and custards, which many people miss if they cannot have them. Of course eating foods with large amounts of sugar in them is never to be recommended but for those who cannot eliminate sugar entirely I am including some recipes containing it.

Custard without milk

Measure the custard powder and sugar and a little cold water into the saucepan in the usual way. Pour the rest of the water boiling straight from the kettle into a measuring jug and float the non-milk creamer on top (about 5 teaspoons to a pint). This will quickly dissolve and can then be poured over the creamed mix and stirred over the heat until it thickens in the usual way. The only noticeable difference is that when cold and set, the top cracks and does not form a thick skin. A liberal scattering of chopped nuts or cherries conceals this on such puddings as trifles.

This milk substitute can also be used in all milk puddings such as rice, sago and tapioca, and is excellent on breakfast cereals, either hot or made the night before and allowed to go cold. We once forgot the creamer on a boat trip and rather than forego breakfast I had the cereal 'black' as well as the coffee: simply with hot water on it. I could hardly detect any difference and continued to eat it this way, even when the creamer was available. After all, non-milk creamers are very much processed foods and I am not suggesting that you should eat them in great abundance. Simply use them as a tool to break the milk habit.

Savoury white sauce

When making white sauce for vegetables, fish and so on, it is not necessary to use milk or the coffee creamer substitute. Heat the margarine and flour with seasoning in the usual way in a saucepan, then pour in a little of the hot water from your vegetable pan or steamed fish, stirring well. Add more boiling water, a little at a time, until the sauce reaches the correct consistency. But don't add any cheese! Use onion or herbs as a flavouring. The sauce will turn white all on its own, just with the vegetable or fish water.

Cream

Once your system is being supplied with only the foods it needs and can tolerate, you will probably not need lashings of cream to take away the acidity of a delicious bowl of fresh fruit salad. You should be able to enjoy fresh, ripe fruit on its own but, if you prefer, you could use custard or blancmange made as above, or coconut cream or soya cream, both of which can be bought in tins, or even mashed banana. Soya milk can be used in all these recipes, but it is expensive and has a distinctive taste which has to be acquired.

Cheese

Cheese is one item that is difficult to replace and is often sadly missed as a snack by many people. Some who are allergic to cow's milk only find they can eat cheese made with goat's milk, and this should be carefully chosen at a good delicatessen and then tested in the diet in the usual way. If you cannot tolerate it, try nut spreads or yeast extract on toast, or make some well-flavoured soya flour cheese.

Soya flour cheese
Melt 110g (4oz) hard set nut oil margarine (obtainable from a health food shop) and fry a chopped onion (and a clove of garlic if liked). Add a liberal sprinkling of your favourite herbs and a teaspoon of turmeric for colour. Now stir in soya flour until it reaches the consistency of thick custard. Cook over a low heat and stir for a few minutes. Then pour into a small mould, such as a margarine tub, and allow to set. This makes a pleasant change with salads or on bread and is rich in protein and high in fibre.

Dried milk powder and whey
Dried milk powder and whey, being almost waste products, are used in all sorts of prepared foods. Many people are under the misapprehension that if they use a low-fat milk powder this is all right. Well, if you just want to lose weight, or to keep to a low-cholesterol diet for the sake of your heart and arteries, then it is fine. But if you suspect you are allergic to dairy produce then it is very likely to be the proteins in the milk which are irritating your system and the only way to test this is also to avoid dried milk and whey. So read the labels on canned, frozen and prepared foods with great care and you will avoid these hazards. Many foods we eat do not have a list of ingredients, so you will have to think twice about foods such as milk chocolate, toffees, prepared desserts and ice cream.

Living Without Wheat Flour and Other Grains

If you have definitely established that wheat flour does not suit you, it could be beneficial to convince your physician that this is so. There are many gluten-free items available on prescription, and it could save you a lot of money to obtain your bread, cakes and biscuits and special flour in this way if you are on free prescriptions. If you cannot convince your doctor of your need for these items, they can be purchased without a prescription at most large dispensaries, but of course are rather expensive. But be warned, they do contain a variety of other ingredients, any one of which may not suit all your requirements, so test each type as a separate food addition. Some are made of cornflour, or just of the starch out of the flour with the gluten removed, and are thus even more processed and refined than ordinary wheat flour and not altogether very satisfying.

It is far better to test out other grains unrelated to wheat to ascertain whether or not you can tolerate any of these and then set about learning to bake with them. It is quite a challenge suddenly to change your entire method of baking, but it can be an enjoyable exercise. You will undoubtedly have your failures as well as successes, but if it is going to help you to feel as much better as I do, it will all be worth while.

The only grain which suits me is rice, but this is good news because there is a great variety of dishes you can make with it. I also use soya, almond, and potato flour, along with soya and rice bran for roughage. Whole ground rice flour is fairly readily obtainable at health food shops and food made with these basic ingredients is filling and nutritious, not to mention cheaper than commercial gluten-free items.

Another grain and flour worth testing for a reaction is buckwheat, which is not related to ordinary wheat. Some people, however, can tolerate cornflour, which is often used to thicken gravies and sauces. Once again, it is vital that you read the labels on canned and prepared foods, because apart from the obvious things to avoid like bread, cakes, pies and biscuits, wheat flour is added to all kinds of other food items in the form of thickeners or rusk, in soups, meat pie fillings, batter coatings, sausages, luncheon meats, and many tinned vegetarian snacks.

Rice flour bread

I have found that the best way to make bread with rice is in the form of a fairly thick batter. Just put all the dry ingredients into a large bowl (in my case about 10 heaped tablespoons rice flour, 2 tablespoons soya flour, 2 tablespoons ground almonds, 2 tablespoons soya bran and $\frac{1}{2}$ teaspoon potassium salt), then rub in about 75g (3oz) vegetable margarine and add sufficient yeast for 675g (1½lb) ordinary flour to make white bread. Mix with sufficient warm water to make a stiff batter, which does not flow smoothly flat when left. Grease and line two medium loaf tins with rice paper or Bakewell (not greaseproof which will not peel off) and two-thirds fill with the mixture. Cover with a polythene bag and leave to rise in a warm place for about an hour, or until it reaches the top of the tin. If you leave it too long, it will collapse again because the mix does not contain gluten to support it. Bake in a hot oven (230°C, 450°F, Gas Mark 8) for about three quarters of an hour or until nicely browned on top.

This bread is rather crumbly, so I have taken to adding a teaspoon of agar agar to the dry mix before adding the warm water and this definitely helps to hold the bread together. It can be used to make toast in the usual way. Potato flour can be substituted for all or part of the rice flour. This holds together better, but is a little dry. When you have tested egg white as a separate item and find you can tolerate it, an egg white added before the water in bread and cakes helps them not to crumble. There is also an egg substitute which can be used for the same purpose. It is called 'Egg Replacer' and, together with several gluten-free items, is available from G.F. Dietary Supplies Ltd, Lowther Road, Stanmore, Middlesex.

Yeast mix fruit cake

Using about half the above basic mixture, add some more vegetable oil, sugar or honey to taste, a teaspoon of mixed spice and plenty of washed dried fruit, cherries and nuts. Allow to rise in the same way, although it will not rise so much, and bake in a foil-lined tin in a hot oven.

Almond Cookies

Almond cookies can be made by combining a cup of ground rice, ½ cup ground almonds, 110g (4oz) vegetable oil or margarine, 50g (2oz) honey or brown sugar and almond essence to taste. Add a little cold water until a thick paste is formed. Shape into flattish cakes and place on rice paper on an oiled baking sheet. Press half an almond into the top of each one if liked. Bake in the top of a hot oven (230°C, 450°F, Gas Mark 8) for about 20 minutes or until just brown. It is very easy to burn these.

With this basic recipe many different flavourings can be achieved with such ingredients as coconut, raisin, date, vanilla, ginger etc.

The basic mix does not make very good pastry as it will not stick together, but it can be used successfully as a crumble topping on top of fruit and baked for a pudding.

Fruit cake not using yeast

Mix up the cake mixture as for yeast mix fruit cake, but without the yeast, or use any variation on rice and potato flour. Combine into a stiff dough with water, then in a cup place a heaped teaspoonful of bicarbonate of soda, a teaspoon of brown sugar and one tablespoon cider vinegar. Beat this mixture thoroughly into the cake mixture and immediately transfer into the baking tin and bake at once in a slower oven (about 180°C, 350°F, Gas Mark 4).

Living Without, or With a Lot Less Sugar

Sugar is a slightly simpler item to abstain from in the practical sense because it is never used to satisfy hunger, more to stimulate our taste buds. By this, I do not mean it is going to be easy to suddenly stop eating sugar – quite the opposite, if you are hooked on lots of it.

Even if you do not have a specific allergic reaction to sugar, in general you would be far better off eating as little as possible. Saccharin and artificial sweeteners are not recommended as there are other question-marks over them. Honey or fructose (sugar refined from fruit) can be used in moderation, but one is really aiming to train the palate to enjoy the natural taste of food without added sweetness. Some people feel they cannot drink a cup of tea or coffee without sugar, but after about a week it is the unanimous opinion of people who have suddenly stopped taking sugar in these drinks that they are far more enjoyable and refreshing without it.

Once again, it is the tinned and prepared foods which are loaded with sugar. Tinned fruit obviously is; not so obvious are the tinned vegetables with sugar added to enhance the flavour. All the prepared puddings, frozen trifles and ice cream, sweets and chocolate are definitely taboo. With a little care it is possible to choose foods with no added sugar, but you will miss the solace of treats of this nature quite badly at first. It is up to you. Are the symptoms you are trying to avoid worse than the deprivation of your favourite chocolates or whatever?

Beware of 'low sugar' labels on cakes and baby foods. Check the actual amounts and, if they are not stated, buy another make or product.

Living Without Salt and Other Individual Items

Eating too much salt can cause high blood pressure in many people, which may bring on disabling strokes and heart disease. It is thus surprising that the need to cut down on salt intake is not more widely publicised, especially as there is a perfectly acceptable substitute condiment based on potassium instead of sodium readily available.

If potassium salt is used in cooking and at the table you are half-way there, but you will have to refrain from eating crisps and peanut-type snacks which rely on salt for their flavour, packeted or tinned soups, meats and so on, which are well laced. Incidentally did you know that bread made without salt is quite tasteless, and so as much as a dessertspoonful is not unknown in a large shop loaf?

The allergic person who has successfully persevered and tracked down more specific items which must be avoided will undoubtedly become used to the idea of finding interesting alternatives, or simply being strong enough to say 'no' when out. Even more difficult is when you are at home alone and perhaps preparing meals for the rest of the family. It is at times like this, when actually handling and smelling the forbidden foods and drinks, that it is all too easy to be tempted to eat some in the privacy of the kitchen, while at the same time carefully serving yourself a suitably different meal. At times like these I sternly remind myself that it is only me that I am fooling and as the whole exercise is for my own benefit it is pretty pointless eating 'naughties' in private!

Make a point of always keeping in stock plenty of treats which you can eat without making yourself feel worse, even if they are usually looked upon as luxuries by the non-allergic members of your household.

– 8 –

Coming To Terms With Rheumatoid Arthritis

As a naive teenager knowing nothing of the potential of diets, or of the dangers of some drugs, I dutifully swallowed the then new wonder cure – steroids. Compared to some people, I was extremely fortunate in that I tolerated them reasonably well and my aches and pains definitely diminished. I am very grateful that these drugs allowed me to live a more normal life, though I was still in too much pain to *enjoy* doing anything. After a while it became obvious I would never be able to take up the career and training originally envisaged, so I reluctantly took a course in shorthand and typing at a little private school run by a marvellously sympathetic lady long past retirement age, whose house was full of hopeful young secretaries and cats.

The cheerful, practical atmosphere and new friends mitigated my bitter disappointment, but the travelling, writing and typing took extreme effort, leaving little energy for any other activities. At the same time, whether due to the steroids, the constant pain or, as I now surmise, to the wrong foods adversely affecting my system, I felt 'ill' most of the time – shaky and weak, rather like having influenza without a cough. This 'fluey' feeling is now known to be common in people with food allergies and it has a detrimental effect on the thinking and reasoning capacity of the victim.

You may think people who are as ill as I have described, and yet try to continue to live normal lives, are in some way brave. But this is not normally the case. When they finally come to terms with the fact there is no more improvement to hope for from the medical profession, there is no alternative but to struggle on, or give up there and then. I did not make many conscious decisions for myself at that time because my mental state was one in which I could not bear to project into the future and I did not have the clarity of reasoning power available to people who are well.

How do you come to terms with the fact that your life is in ruins and that you have been unfortunate enough to get a disease which will not go away? In most cases the illness starts slowly and creeps up on you. Many a patient has spent years continuing to work uncomplainingly whilst taking increasing doses of painkilling drugs. Eventually having to give up employment and unwillingly accept a large fall in income means their standard of living takes a drastic change for the worse. When the victim is also the family breadwinner, the result can be catastrophic. Often there is no hope of meeting mortgage payments and the home has to be sold – with the family moving either to a smaller house or to council-subsidised accommodation.

If, as is more often the case, the disease strikes the woman of the house while she is not employed outside the home, but working full-time bringing up her children and managing the home, the results are not so apparent, nor dramatic. She simply cuts down on additional activities – usually the fun things like outings and sports – in order to use her diminishing energies caring for her family to the best of her remaining ability. She cannot usually claim any form of sickness benefit but also has to forget any ideas she may have treasured of resuming her career once the children are old enough not to demand so much attention.

Thus an army of sick married women is provided for, if not actually nursed, within the family and consequently does not appear in any statistics of unemployed and unemployable.

Could this contribute to the relative lack of resources devoted to researching this disease, which is certainly not glamorous enough to attract much publicity for fund-raising or elaborate projects to publicise the plight of the victims? If rheumatoid arthritis resulted after a few years in death and not just in a life-sentence of the end of all enjoyment, perhaps there would be more interest in prevention.

For my part, I became a reasonably competent, if slow, secretary and worked as such for a few years until the constant banging away at a typewriter had caused my shoulders, arms and hands to become so painful that full-time work had to be given up. Quite apart from this physical side of things, I also disliked intensely the monotony, waste and pettiness of office life and yearned for a more adventurous, outdoor existence, presumably as does many a fitter office girl.

I am writing the book I wish I had been able to read all those years ago and which I firmly believe would have saved me years of pain and enabled me to do many of the things I wished to do. However, if someone had told me or my parents early on in my illness that I could help myself by drastically changing my eating habits, we would probably not have believed them. All our early education and habits are so ingrained that it is extremely difficult to change them. Not only is this the case, but we seem to go along to our medical practitioners with a rather pathetic faith in their ability to make us better. This doctor/patient relationship is, of necessity, based on an often despairing hope on the side of the patient and relatives, and a genuine desire to help, tempered with knowledge of the harsh reality about the limitations of medicine, on the part of the doctor. After all, he or she is only a caring human being, who has opted to accept some of the awesome responsibility for other people's lives.

While it is true that members of the medical profession undergo extensive general training over a wide field and that modern science is coming up with new ideas all the while, the time has come to ask ourselves whether we are expecting too much, not only of general practitioners but specialists as well. Should not society as a whole and individuals in particular accept more of the responsibility for their own positive health and not have so much blind faith in the medical profession putting everything right with a few different pills or operations?

When the chips are really down, after the medics have tried everything at their disposal, and the patient is still not recovering sufficiently, the only person who really cares is the patient. Apart from loving parents and spouses, who may sometimes be able to help in many ancillary ways, it is the conscious effort of each individual to help his or herself which is all-important.

I did not want to be in any sense a rebel. I had no ambition to write articles, or study diets in the sort of detail given here. It has been forced upon me by circumstances. First of all my aim was to help myself, and once that was successful beyond all hopes, I resolved to assist other people who are in pain and try and save them years of misery.

I would have much prefered to have a local doctor whom I could consult at each stage of my dietary progress for help, advice, and most of all confirmation and encouragement that what I was doing was along the right lines. I felt I needed advice in case vital elements were being missed on such a restricted diet and at times it needed all my willpower to continue. Eventually, some time after I had discovered my worst allergens, I saw a request for assistance with case histories from a research group. Naturally I wrote them of my success and was fortunate indeed to be able to correspond to this day with a doctor specialising in clinical ecology who has helped and encouraged me greatly.

We must work towards passing the initial treatment of allergic patients back to ordinary doctors. Allergy is such a widespread phenomenon that it would save a tremendous amount of pain and suffering from a diversity of illnesses if patients were to be routinely tested for staple food allergies first, before being placed on drugs or having their symptoms treated by something as major as surgery.

These tests, although undoubtedly time-consuming, require no expensive equipment or highly qualified medics. Trained technicians and nurses in a local unit could treat patients in a controlled environment and within days establish whether the trouble was allergy-based. Within three weeks they could identify the major allergens and educate patients sufficiently for them to continue to be well at home.

Even if this type of investigation took a month, it would be cheaper than many of the present unsatisfactory methods of treating the disease, and would be far less painful and alarming for the patients, who should then be able to resume their previous lifestyle with every expectancy of remaining fit and active if they are disciplined enough to maintain the suitable diet individually worked out for them.

As it is likely to be many years before such treatment is available, you will probably be trying this approach at home. In that case, please do not suddenly decrease or stop taking any medication which has been prescribed for you. Change nothing but your diet, or you will not be able to tell which change is affecting your health. If, after a while, you feel very much better, it is usually safe to lower your dose of or stop taking pain-killers altogether, but do please consult your doctor before decreasing the dosage of any other tablets. If you have any doubts at all, consult your doctor before you begin your experiments.

I would be more than willing to assist any area health authority or specialist rheumatology unit to set up an experiment, with a view to adopting a new approach towards the diet of their patients in conjunction with orthodox treatments. One of the advantages of the controlled diet approach is that it can be instituted at any time in the patient's treatment with no other drastic changes, until benefits begin to be enjoyed, when tablets and injections can diminish in a controlled fashion. A satisfactory position is eventually reached of balance between diet and less tablets, physiotherapy and other treatments.

– 9 –

Using Your Own Symptoms To Help Discover Which Foods Upset Your System

There is a whole set of illnesses, symptoms or inconveniences – call them what you like – from which many people suffer which are gradually becoming recognised as indicators of an allergic condition. These include persistent indigestion, bloating or swelling of the stomach, constipation, day-long fatigue and desire to sleep longer than usual, sleeplessness or hyperactivity, dark rings under the eyes even when rested, a high pulse rate which can be felt in the chest, persistent catarrh, coughs or colds which do not clear up, spots, headaches, frequent and urgent passing of urine, sudden mood changes, depression, anxiety – this list could go on and on with the many modern afflictions which sometimes become severe enough to take us to our GP.

The doctor is in a dilemma. Maybe he knows many of these ills are self-inflicted, but it will not improve his relationship with his patients if he tells them so. Anyway, he has not the time to go into their emotional, environmental and dietary background; all too often he will simply prescribe some tablets to suppress the worst of the symptoms. This may help the patient to cope in the short-term, but it does nothing to sort out his real problems – in fact it may even compound them.

In Chapter One I described the palpitations, or racing heart or pulse rate, which I had when my rheumatoid arthritis was in its early stages. This persisted until, twenty years later, I traced my allergies and eliminated the foods which were causing them and the resultant pain. Goodness knows how this has affected my heart and circulatory system, but it has now accepted a slower lifestyle without further complaint. I still cannot take any prolonged activity without a rest, which is maybe one result of the unnecessary wear and tear formerly experienced by my cardiovascular system.

Ancillary symptoms can be useful in gauging your reaction to the various foods. The pulse rate reacts quite quickly to the food eaten and this phenomenon can be used to judge if and how badly you are allergic to the various items. Headaches and catarrh, flushes and dizziness can come and go quickly too, and all such symptoms should be noted in your chart.

I suggest you choose a time when you are feeling reasonably well just before a meal. Sit down quietly for a few minutes so your pulse rate is not raised by recent exercise and have a notebook and pencil handy. Now take your pulse. This is done by placing two fingers of one hand lightly on your other wrist just above the inner side of the thumb. Do not use the thumb to feel your wrist as there is a pulse in the thumb which could mislead you. Move the fingers gently about until you feel the pulse beat. In some people whose wrists are deformed with arthritic growth it may be quite difficult to find, or indeed you may not be able to manoeuvre one hand suitably to the other to do this. In either case it may be easier for you to find the pulse on the temple or in the neck. Those in the neck lie either side of the windpipe and beat quite strongly as they are closer to the heart than the wrist.

The usual pulse rate of most normal, healthy adults is 70–80 beats per minute, babies having a higher rate. (Athletes often have a lower pulse rate, which is a great asset, because when they speed their heartbeat up during prolonged exertion it does not have to work as hard as other people's). Note down the rate you have established, together with the time, and how you are feeling. I found it handy to use my food diary for this and just made myself an extra column.

To complete your test, consume a usual-sized portion of the food or drink under test. Remember, just one item at a time, so a glass of milk would be fine, but not a cup of coffee with milk and sugar. Black coffee or tea with no sugar would be suitable, or a portion of potatoes, peas, plain fruit, meat, fish or mushrooms. Take your pulse again immediately after eating and note it down. Then take it again in twenty minutes time, then again forty minutes and one hour after eating. If the rate goes up after the meal you should suspect that particular food. The more rapidly the pulse rises, the more seriously you should suspect it.

The pulse rate will probably return to normal once the food has been digested. Normal for most allergic people is usually pretty high. Mine was almost always over 100. It is now mostly at 80 but naturally varies with exertion, excitement or if I eat the wrong foods. It is most interesting and satisfying to watch the pulse rate on your chart gradually come down and settle at a more sedate pace as you one by one eliminate all the things which were causing it to race. Once you have tested several foods which do not raise your pulse rate or cause other unpleasant symptoms, you can put these on your 'safe' list and continue to eat them whilst testing different items at the same meal. So although this method can take a long time, it is only for the first few days that it is rather inconvenient. In fact, some people become so adept at the method that they can casually take their pulse under the table when invited out to dinner and test a new food which they suspect may not suit them, thus furthering science without offending their hosts!

At the same time as noting your pulse rate you should record your other symptoms. These two indicators taken together should give you a fairly accurate picture of what to eat and what to leave strictly alone. Occasionally you will get a normal pulse reading but a reaction of increased symptoms in other directions, in which instance this should be counted as an adverse reaction. If you are not sure about any particular item, test it again at another time in a different combination and circumstances, but do try to keep coherent notes, or your efforts will be wasted. Memory alone is just not accurate enough.

Should you get a bad dose of pain and illness following one of your tests, a heaped teaspoon of bicarbonate of soda in water will help to neutralize the acids formed and clear the system. It is preferable not to try any more experiments until the effect of a bad one has entirely worn off. It could be the next day or even three days later.

You may have read in the press about blood tests which can be carried out to see if people are allergic to various foods. These are popular in America and are called cytotoxic tests. To put it simply, a sample of your blood is individually mixed with up to 170 different food samples. The blood cells react in differing ways and under the microscope it is possible to tell which foods have had an adverse effect on the blood cells. As you can imagine, such a labour-intensive, skilled test is expensive. I believe these have now been imported into the UK and are available privately. They may seem a very convenient way to discover your allergens without all that effort on your part, but unfortunately these blood tests are not as accurate as one would hope. Neither are scratch or prick tests.

It is also possible to have a sample of hair tested for past mineral levels and levels of toxic metals. These need to be correctly interpreted by an expert who can then prescribe suitable supplements and actions to clear abnormal levels of lead and so on.

Some NHS doctors do have allergy skin-testing kits which they can be persuaded to use on patients whom they suspect may have an allergy. These test for reactions to various inhalants, dusts, moulds, mites, etc, but do not test for the sort of staple food allergy which is more important to arthritics. Anyway, no one yet seems to have convinced the NHS that rheumatoid arthritis and many other serious diseases may be allergy-based. Thus, unfortunately, it all comes back to you, the person with the problem, sorting it out yourself at home with very little, if any, encouragement from your medical advisors, or even with frosty disapproval and disbelief in some cases. However, it is your life, so take it into your own hands and try to do something about it. You have my assurance that reasonably juggling about with your diet cannot possibly make you worse, and the odds are heavily in favour of it making you feel a great deal better.

Have a serious try and, if you succeed, tell your doctor about it in the most diplomatic way you know of, just in case he gradually becomes convinced enough to suggest it to some other patient who may not know of this self-help therapy. Doctors are only human and I heard of a case where a doctor's own child had been virtually cured of asthma by dietary means. Yet he still did not recommend this treatment to the mother of a similarly afflicted young patient because he felt she might not believe him. Meanwhile she independently read of and applied an elimination diet with similar success. Her feelings on reporting back to the doctor and finding the cure was already familiar to him can only be imagined.

I should also mention sub-lingual tests. 'Sub-lingual' means 'under the tongue' and these tests consist of introducing under the tongue, in controlled experiments, minute quantities of various foods which have been ground up and stirred into water. These are fully described in books purely about allergies and can be a fairly quick way of finding reactions, but arthritics' pain reactions tend to be slower, so to us they are perhaps not so useful.

It is quite possible to conduct any of these tests alone at home and many people have done so successfully, but if you have a supportive spouse, parent or friend to encourage and assist you or even just take an interest, the whole thing becomes more fun and can strengthen your resolve to continue, as there is no doubt you will need plenty of determination not to lapse into indulgent, comfortable, quick and easy eating habits again, particularly in the early days before you feel much benefit. It is even better if several people with similar problems can get together and share notes, recipes and experiences.

Twenty-five years ago, the advice for arthritics was to

exercise in order to keep joints moving to their full capacity. Although I enquired of several different rheumatologists, I could never obtain any exact guidance as to the amount and type of exercise which could safely be undertaken. People vary greatly in their capabilities and reaction to pain, so perhaps no hard and fast rules are possible. Also advocated then and still today were painkillers, drugs to suppress swelling, gold injections, splints, hydrotherapy and social gatherings to cheer patients up. Research is being undertaken into possible virus causes, or replacement of existing strong and expensive drugs with new ones, but not enough priority is being given by the medical profession to research into the effect of the food we eat upon serious long-term illness. Naturally I feel rather sad about this because I know the benefits which can be derived from such dietary control.

After all, the National Health Service can always make use of more money to spend on health care. Arthritic patients must cost an enormous amount to care for throughout their long and painful lives. For instance I was hospitalised for one month on average every two years, and consumed many drugs, until I stopped eating all the wrong (for me) foods. Since then I have attended as an outpatient to see the consultant for a few minutes interview at longer and longer intervals over the years. He is obviously pleased to see that I do not need so much help from him, enquires about the diet I have mentioned, but does not comment. For many years now I have never felt so well in all my adult life, except on those rare occasions when I slip up and eat something I should not.

A recent example springs to mind of how this can happen accidentally. I make all my own bread and cakes using mainly rice flour as I am allergic to wheat and other grains. This, together with abstaining from the other items I have discovered I should not eat, has succeeded in keeping me very well for years now, but recently I gradually began to feel the return of many of my long-forgotten aches, plus listlessness and indigestion. Frantically I searched my soul (and pantry) to try to discover what I was eating which could possibly be causing the trouble. Eventually I remembered I had purchased a supply of rice flour from a different health food shop that was whiter in colour and made better bread which did not crumble as much.

Quickly, I obtained some of the genuine rice flour from my usual supplier (who rather inconveniently happens to be twenty miles from my home), made some new bread and over several weeks began to feel better again. I have no way of knowing what was in the suspect flour, or any way of proving to the shopkeeper the pain and distress it caused me.

On another occasion I purchased some potato flour which was labelled 'farina' on the package. The proprietor of the shop assured me the product was invoiced as potato flour, but the effect it had on me when turned into a cake told me it had much else in it too. It was only then that I looked up 'farina' in the dictionary: 'Flour or meal of corn, nuts, or starchy roots; powdery substance; starch.'

It would make life a great deal easier for allergic people, who are still not always sympathetically received in shops if *all* contents were clearly indicated on the wrapper. So be warned by these examples of my experiences and shop even more carefully.

You have to want to improve your health as well as have the discipline to do so. At the time I changed my life by discovering my allergens, some of my joints were approaching the stage of that last admission of defeat by conventional methods: joint replacement. This would have meant horrifically large operations to eventually achieve less pain and more mobility in one joint only, with the disease continuing to flourish in all other respects. Nowadays, although my joints which were so nearly ready for operations are still limited in their movement, there is no pain when I am at rest, and very little in ordinary use, but they do protest if I abuse them. Instead of continuing to deteriorate, the range of movement has actually increased very, very gradually and the appearance of most joints, particularly wrists and hands, is unbelievably improved. On casual acquaintance, most people have no idea I have rheumatoid arthritis for at the worst I appear rather clumsy in certain movements.

In the days when I was very stiff and experiencing a lot of pain, I conscientiously exercised to the limit of every joint movement as often as I remembered each morning. I agree with all the doctors and books that this is essential to maintain as much movement as possible. But at the same time, extent of movement was diminishing due to the pain and lack of muscle power, plus physical restriction. After relaxing the muscles and soothing the pain in a hot bath it is possible to extend the range by pushing an arm gently further up against the wall, or kneeling down and pressing your weight to force your knees to bend a little more. Or get a friend or relative to lift the weight of the limb and gently move it for you. Don't overdo it, though.

I will describe a few of the errors I made in case it helps you to avoid similar mistakes and damage which cannot be repaired. Some of my worst joint damage has been caused by continuing to do things which were hurting just too much. Bashing away for long hours at a manual typewriter I feel was the cause of my wrists deteriorating, and my right elbow, which always disliked any small gripping motions in that hand, like knitting or crochet, was permanently injured when trying to assist in a building operation by cutting out too much sheet metal with tin shears. A knee suffered the same fate when I walked too far through soft mud in borrowed boots which were too large. The effort of pulling them up out of the suction of the mud at every step was just too much. When it was too late I realised I would have been better off removing them and going barefoot. (Even better not to have missed the tide and gone aground!)

On the other hand, I always did and still do occasionally enjoy extending the range of manual tasks I can achieve – like digging the garden over a little at a time, going up ladders to paint or fix things, sailing, driving, woodwork and so on. But now I am older and a little wiser I usually have the sense to stop when I should. Therefore my recommendations on exercise are to do as much as you can of the things you enjoy, but not to the extent of constant pressure or wear on any particular joint. Stop at once if it begins to complain more than usual.

The best exercise is that taken unnoticed during an activity which you enjoy and preferably has some useful outcome. I cannot recommend a regular regime of specific exercises other than a complete range of joint movement each day, because most people soon become bored with them. You may perhaps enjoy the social outing of a keep-fit class, but many arthritics have too much restriction in movement to partake fully and feel self-conscious of ugly limbs in such company. This is a pity, because the same feelings often prevent us from enjoying the best exercise there is for arthritics – swimming, or at least splashing around in the water. Apart from limited hydrotherapy at the hospital, most arthritics do not have the opportunity to feel the bliss of moving freely in warm water with the weight taken off those painful joints and not so much muscle power required to lift arms and legs. Just walking about with your weight supported by the buoyancy of the water helps to strengthen muscles and reminds them how to move properly and what their function is. If you are able to swim, this is an ideal way of exercising the whole body gently without putting stress on any one part. Why not pluck up your courage and get an able-bodied friend to accompany you to the local heated pool to give you confidence and help support you if necessary. Many pools reserve a quiet period for disabled people. I am sure you will really enjoy yourself, but I have to admit that weather permitting I prefer the relative privacy of the sea, even if it is rather colder.

Another enjoyable and beneficial form of exercise for those who can still manage it is cycling. Again this can be gentle exercise which does not entail all the weight going onto knees and feet. Once I started to feel better and had a little more strength and confidence, and had lost my dizziness, I was given as a present an old-fashioned, sit-up-and-beg bicycle. After a few tentative and rather wobbly tries I really enjoyed spinning along the quiet country roads near to home. I could not get to the village shops, 1½ miles away, without several stops for a rest, not because of pain, but because of lack of stamina from enforced inactivity, but was gradually extending my range when the bicycle was stolen. Sad to say it was considered a bit of a time-consuming luxury, it being quicker to go shopping by car, so the bicycle was never replaced.

Of late I do not do many conscious exercises, just a good stretch now and then when I have been sitting too long at the typewriter, or lain awkwardly at night. I rely on everyday activities which can now be carried out with so much more enthusiasm to keep me mobile and it certainly seems to work. I do make a special effort to walk properly and not to stoop.

As in most things, exercise is a personal preference and as long as you take a certain amount every day, gradually increasing your range, and do not over-stress any joints by pounding away with too much of one type of work or play, I am sure you will derive the benefits of greater strength, mobility, general stamina and well-being.

– 10 –

Why We Have Food Allergies

There is not much agreement amongst professionals as to why so many more people are becoming allergic to various substances.

One theory is that there were always the same number of people suffering, but that their symptoms were not correctly diagnosed.

Another is that the food we eat and the atmosphere we live in at home, at work or even out of doors, is so polluted with modern chemicals that it makes us more prone to allergies.

It is easy to see why workers who handle strong chemicals, or women who do the laundry with harsh detergents, should sometimes get an allergic rash on their hands. Sprayers of insecticides and herbicides risk inhaling these products as do the victims situated on the field's edge who receive an accidental dose, particularly from aerial sprayers who cannot, by their very nature, be as accurate as one would wish. A wise headmistress of a country school once mentioned to me that a bout of sickness amongst her pupils, called food poisoning by the local doctor, appeared to coincide with the spraying season each spring.

But what of the spray which makes its mark and actually lands on the crops as intended? It does an efficient job in killing the greenfly, blackfly and other pests, no doubt along with the ladybirds and other allies of the farmer. Other sprays also clear the field of competitive weeds, as is witnessed by the unbroken acres of shimmering wheat with never a poppy or dog-daisy to spoil the view. A few wild flowers might manage to survive along the edges and roadsides to delight us. A couple of years ago a local field caused traffic jams as cars were brought to a halt by the sight of a tree and hedgelined meadow of corn dotted copiously with flaming red poppies. Cameras clicked non-stop to record this unusual sight, yet until recent years it was common. I never did discover whether the treat was a happy accident on the part of the farmer, or carefully nurtured for the background to certain TV commercials. Whatever the cause, it gave a great deal of pleasure and it would be interesting to know its effect on the yield of wheat compared to neighbouring 'barren' prairies.

One wonders what happens to all these chemicals after they have performed the initial task intended. They can't just disappear. Does a certain amount remain in the soil, or is it left on the food? Much of it is washed out of the soil and into the watercourses, eventually entering our rivers and destroying the fish and other wildlife.

As mentioned earlier, I love the countryside and am fortunate to be able to live in a beautiful part of England, but here I can see the effects of intensive farming methods at first hand. Twenty years ago the local rivers and lakes were full of fish and water birds, living quite happily alongside hundreds of holiday-makers in the summer months. The water remained clear and productive, apart from becoming churned up by the propellers and wash waves of over-fast motorboats. Amateur fishermen caught plenty of fish and put them back. Those more expert fishermen, the herons and other fish-eating birds, flourished.

Gradually boat traffic increased with the boom in holidays. At great cost, the authorities, concerned about the quality of the water, ruled that toilets must no longer be pumped straight overboard, but go to storage tanks to be emptied at boat yards. Where the waste then goes to underground may not be so clear. Even if a main sewer was available to the remote locations involved, main sewers in my area have the habit of emptying their contents back into the river somewhere else, maybe somewhat treated, but now containing even more of the harmful toxic chemicals which have to be added to the boat storage tanks. The enrichment of the water from that source was not too harmful in its original form, although unpleasant for swimmers in the more populous areas.

Sink waste was allowed to continue to be drained overboard into the water. Ironically although this was aesthetically more acceptable to the holidaymakers, the phosphates in the detergents it contained are far more harmful and contribute greatly to the eutrophication (over-enrichment) of the water. Town sewage outfalls naturally contain large quantities of phosphate, although one small local works near me has reluctantly installed a stripping system on an experimental basis.

However, even with all this expense and inconvenience to the boat trade, the water quality continued to deteriorate with whole rivers now turning a murky green colour which, together with the muddy sediment, shaded out the advantageous, oxygen-producing water plants. This green hue is caused by countless billions of algae which multiply rapidly because the water is over-enriched with nitrates and phosphates, mainly from human wastes and farmers' fertilisers which leach out of the fields into dykes which are in turn pumped into the main rivers and lakes. The increased use of fertilisers comes about as more and more ancient grazing marshes are deep drained and ploughed for sowing with arable crops.

The total ecology of any given area is complex, with changes creeping up on it until breaking point is reached. Our local breaking point came when the navigation authority deepened a channel through a lake situated near the sea. At the same time, local farmers were digging deep drainage dykes to convert the grazing marshes to arable land. In both cases, the underlying salt-water table was reached, and salt thus mingled with the fresh-water system.

The brackish, fertiliser-enriched water provided just the

right conditions for the alga Prymnesium to bloom and multiply rapidly during a period of bright sunny weather. Came a few days of duller weather and the water could support them no longer, with catastrophic effects. In dying the Prymnesium released a poison which in turn killed every fish species in the whole system. They eventually floated to the surface and lay rotting in their thousands along the lee banks, in places nose to tail. Eels, which can put up with a lot of pollution, were seen leaving the water to wriggle across paths and grassland in an effort to escape the poisonous river.

The area has now in part healed its wounds, returning to a pale shadow of its former glory, but the main causes of the trouble have not been removed. Thus now and again the few fish which have misguidedly swum in from other areas die in minor toxic algae blooms, while nothing really flourishes in the murky waters. The local university have carried out expensive studies to see what can be done. They published their initial findings. 'The seagulls roosting at night in large numbers on one of the more extensive lakes were responsible for polluting the water'! The deepening of the inland drainage dykes continues, with more and more grazing marshes being converted to cereal.

This whole sad story can be almost directly likened to the eco-system of a human being. It is possible to pour food that is too rich or unsuitable in large quantities into yourself for many years with hardly any apparent ill-effects, until one day another food, or a combination of stressful circumstances such as examinations, pregnancy, bereavement, an unconnected infection or perhaps loss of employment can trigger off similar cataclysmic happenings to you. If you can later track down the circumstances and put your eco-system to rights again, Nature is a wonderful healer and will take over to put things in order again: maybe not always 100%, but as in my case and many others, so much so that you will be happy to stay on a restricted diet if it will keep you feeling so much better and lessen the suffering.

Left to themselves wild animals are very fussy eaters. It is no good taking domestic or farm animals as an example because we tend to change their eating habits to suit our convenience. But consider the herbivores: grazing deer and goats, wildebeest, buffalo, moose and so on. They prefer new green shoots of a limited variety, but will eat dry grass and other vegetation during a drought. Their whole system is geared to deal with this kind of diet and very fit, lithe and energetic they appear to be. Preying on these vegetarians are the carnivores: the meat-eating cat family, wolves, eagles, who have a very different digestive system but cope equally successfully. In between are the omnivores, or animals who eat whatever they can find, be it animal or vegetable. Man falls into this latter category along with the apes and other primates from whom we are said to be descended. The wilder members of these relations continue to eat mainly green vegetables and rather fussily at that, choosing the tender growing tips which contain more protein, plus nice ripe fruits and maybe the odd bird's egg or small reptile if available.

If we captured such an animal for a zoo and fed it a typical Western human diet, it would probably become very ill or die. In fact, feeding-time at the zoo is a good object lesson to us. In order to maintain the health of their charges the keepers study carefully the background and original diet of each member and then copy it. They provide raw fish for the penguins and otters; whole raw meat for the lions; bamboo for the pandas; whole mice or chicks for the birds of prey and snakes; seeds for the finches and so on. We occasionally hear or read reports about popular zoo inmates which have become ill and are then 'cured' when someone realises foods such as monkey food and eggs do not keep a panda healthy, or that monkeys and pet dogs should not be fed human treats of sweets or even beer.

We could do a similar back-to-nature exercise for ourselves, except that our natural origins are too distant to remember or know with any certainty. But let us work on the things we do know. Being related to the apes, we were probably hunter/gatherers in much the same way, eating young green leaves, fruit, roots, nuts, occasionally supplemented with eggs and small animals, fish and insects. All this food was obviously growing wild and naturally. Plenty of gentle, regular exercise was required to gather it. More vigorous exercise was required to flee from predators and stay alive.

Much later in our evolution we became organised hunters and are often portrayed by historians as fur-clad savages eating mainly meat in caves. The more primitive tribes left in the world today demonstrate the inaccuracy of this picture, for they still exist on a mainly vegetable diet with hunting only bringing in a rare treat of meat, particularly with those tribes which do not have guns. Even when they graduate from hunting and gathering to gardening for survival, the produce is mainly vegetable, such as sweet potato, maize, rice, millet, sago, and potato, depending on the part of the world and climate. The domestic animals tend to be kept as status symbols, only to be slaughtered and eaten at special feasts or bartered for brides.

Another difference between the primitive diet and ours is that the food had to be eaten whole. There were not the machinery or techniques, time and labour to refine grain by removing the husks or finely milling it, then sieving and bleaching the flour. Instead, the whole grain was ground or pounded by hand each day and cooked fresh. Obviously it had no contamination from fertiliser or poisonous chemicals. Food tended to be rather scarce and difficult to store, so people were prevented from over-eating except in times of glut. Variety was forced upon them during changing seasons. It was not possible to eat the same favourite food every day direct from the supermarket or home freezer. If a certain fish were not in season, or crop ready for gathering, you waited with eager anticipation for its arrival.

Animals were grazed cheaply on the untouched wild pastures, so the milk and cheese produced would also be uncontaminated. Refined sugar was unknown, wild honey must have been popular, but not available in sufficient quantities to produce the almost universal sweet tooth of modern times.

Therefore, as well as avoiding the foods which you now find

you have become allergic to, I am also seriously suggesting that you try to eat as much natural food as possible. Have a much reduced portion of whatever animal protein still suits you, and eat plenty of fresh vegetables and salad from as good an unadulterated source as possible, and any grains or flour which your system can tolerate which are of the whole ground variety and have not been subjected to cosmetic processing and additives. Strictly avoid all junk food, sugary drinks and stimulants. Fresh fish is a better source of animal protein than any kind of meat, for it is the only kind which is still hunted wild and not overfed and chemically injected.

Maybe it is because fruit and vegetables just have to be eaten with most of their goodness and fibre still in them that they are so much better for us than the flour, sugar, meat and milk products we have discussed. It is best to eat most vegetables raw, cooking the rest quickly in a pressure cooker or lightly stir-frying them in the oriental way in order to retain as many of the minerals and vitamins as possible: they can be destroyed by too much heat. That great British staple, the potato, is very enjoyable baked in its scrubbed jacket as an alternative to the eternal mashed, fried and roasted varieties, for the skin contains much of the flavour and fibre.

Whilst on the subject of eating a generally healthier diet, I must mention salt. It is now accepted by most authorities that over-consumption of common salt (sodium salt) is a common cause of high blood pressure. Controlled tests have been carried out where half a group ate salt as usual and half were given a potassium salt substitute (this is available from health food shops). The blood pressure of the latter group fell appreciably with no other treatment. It is also believed that common sodium salt causes fluid retention problems as well as a higher incidence of strokes.

– 11 –

Positive Health And Sensible Eating

Milk

On first thinking about it, you may feel that milk is one of the purest and most nourishing natural foods obtainable. Well so it is – for calves! It is designed specifically to nourish and quickly build up young calves into adult cows or bulls. Once they are weaned they would receive very short shrift from Mama if they tried to continue to get their daily pinta into old age. In other words, not only is it unnatural for us humans to drink the milk of another species, but we should ask ourselves whether there are any other animals once they are weaned from their mother's milk which continue to have milk products on the menu at all.

At the time of writing, there is a welcome return to encouraging mothers to breast-feed their babies. At last it is being recognised that cow's milk is not suitable for the digestive system of a newborn human – even if moderated in various ways – however good it might be for the calf.

Particularly sensitive youngsters, even though breast-fed by their mother, are still made ill by the effects of their particular allergen coming through the mother. If the mother can trace the food item causing the screaming, rashes, asthma or whatever, and then abstain from eating it herself, the baby will begin to thrive. As there are more and more articles in the press and news items on radio and television about this, one would hope that more attention would be given to this aspect of treating obviously unhappy, if not ill, babies. Yet still we hear of desperate parents who have a child who screams all day and almost all night from birth and continues to be miserable to 3 or 5 years old, before by chance they are put on the right dietary lines by reading an article or meeting someone who recognises allergies and can help them. It seems unbelievable that this simple expedient is rarely used by doctors and staff in the NHS for it is quick and effective as well as cheap.

One simple reason why it is often cow's milk that is the culprit with babies and toddlers is because they have been fed this, and very little else, if not right from birth, then from being weaned from their mother. At least it makes it simpler to examine their diet and eliminate possible irritants. The result can be quite astounding, as in the case of one little girl in our home village, who at 18 months was transformed from a screaming embarrassment to her parents into a happy, well-behaved model daughter who is a joy to have around, as long as you make sure well-intentioned friends and relatives do not give her any treats with the wrong foodstuffs in them. On these accidental occasions she reverts to her former tantrums and upset tummy, until the 'poisons' work their way out of her system again.

In these days of high production and cost efficiency down on the farm as well as in the factory, every effort is put into increasing the milk yield of the herd, and so cows are selectively bred to have huge udders, and scientifically fed just the right amount of additional expensive food pellets to enable them to produce maximum yields. They receive a high standard of veterinary attention; calves are removed as early as possible so the precious milk can be channelled into profit. Cows are frequently kept in sheds to be fed harvested grass, grain and silage, rather than allowed to roam the field, lest they trample and foul some of the growing food.

The Milk Marketing Board has a surplus and uses advertising to reduce it. Customers are told how good milk is for them, how it is mean not to have butter instead of the more healthy vegetable margarine, that cheese is excellent value and delicious, cream is 'naughty but nice'; and with flavoured milks children are encouraged to imbibe even more milk.

In addition, we pay farmers grants on the cost of converting unsuitable land, be it draining irreplaceable marshland or ploughing ancient heaths, in order to grow grain to feed to cattle. In some cases we also pay landowners *not* to despoil sites of special interest and beauty to compensate their farmers who are prevented from joining in the bonanza. Why not have a planning permission system for the countryside, similar to that in built up areas? After all there is no compensation if you are not allowed to build a factory in a residential area. This would at least protect what little unspoiled countryside remains. But better still, let us return to a sane system where local small farmers, whose families have known and loved the area for generations, produce just sufficient for our needs and their living wages, without all the costs of marketing. A good deal of unnecessary organisation and transportation could be avoided.

I am sorry if I seem to over-emphasise the bad side of too much milk in the diet, but I lost 20 of what could have been the best years of my life due to this substance, so the more I see of the futile politics of it, the more upset I feel. Although Common Market policy has belatedly changed to try to control milk production with a quota system, insufficient is done to warn of the dangers of too much dairy produce in the diet. I can well understand how the milk story had its beginnings in more benevolent times. It was seen as a rich source of protein, vitamins and nourishment for underfed children in city slums, when poverty and rickets were a reality. Cheap or free milk for nursing mothers and babies long ago helped to cure these deficiencies, but the practice continues today, along with a folk-lore image of milk being good, if not indispensable, for the health. We all forget that at one time cow's milk was a main carrier of tuberculosis.

Well I, and many others like me, am able to tell you the other side of the story. Not only can it be bad for most of us if taken in excessive amounts, but milk can have a positively harmful effect on a lesser proportion of the population who happen to be allergic to it as I have tried to describe.

My criticisms of cow's milk so far have been directed against the excess use of it in the Western diet, but regrettably there are other reasons to suspect it. First is the 'good' husbandry which enables each cow to produce more milk daily than nature intended. Most people know that for flavour and goodness you do not choose huge, overgrown fruit and vegetables. These are for record seekers at the horticultural shows. First choice for eating is medium-sized, preferably organically grown produce, which has withstood the sun and wind and in some cases frost as well. Generally speaking, only then is the full taste and goodness present. I do not see why it should be different with cattle. If you feed a cow an unnaturally rich diet and cosset it too much, might not its udder be compared to the champion marrow at the local show?

A second, more serious cause for concern is the routine injection of calves with antibiotics and drugs to make them grow quickly and keep infections at bay. They also have dubious elements in their food. Cattle are grazing animals and not strictly grain eaters, nor seekers of silage and fish meal for that matter. Left to themselves, they would have a very thin diet in winter which would give their milk production a rest between calves. They would also take a lot of exercise to burn off some of the surplus fat which now gets left in the meat. Traces of all these elements can come through into the milk which we drink and the meat we eat to have a cumulative effect on our health.

Much time and effort is spent on promoting the fast growth of farm animals and poultry, so they can start producing milk or eggs or be turned into butchers' meat at the earliest date. Cattle can put on two pounds weight a day and be slaughtered within a year. Pigs are killed for meat in six months, growing five times faster than the wild boar from which they are descended. Do the hormones used for this purpose linger in the animal products when we eat them? Do the additives then go on to act adversely on our bodies? I raise these questions because our young people appear to be reaching puberty at an earlier and earlier age and to be experiencing more difficulties at this time. Although there has been a trend for humans to increase in height over the centuries, the latest generations appear to be growing disproportionately taller than previous generations. This especially applies to young girls who are mortified to find they are too tall to be able to wear the off-the-peg fashionable clothes and shoes which are so important to them during their teens.

By the nature of things, farm animals very often do not fully grow up and never grow old, so we cannot know the effects in later life of the growth-accelerating and muscle-promoting drugs they are given as youngsters. But we humans all hope and expect to grow old, so it might be beneficial to know for certain if the incidental hormone treatment we receive in this way is detrimental to our health in the longterm. The increasing incidence of painful periods, pre-menstrual tension and extreme symptoms suffered during the change of life by too many women could, I believe, have their origins in the eating of too much contaminated animal produce.

Wheat and Other Arable Products

A similar scenario applies to certain other aspects of agriculture, particularly wheat and other grains, too much of which is fed to animals. It is a grand excuse for the farming administration to be able to claim 'we are feeding the nation' as if they are doing it out of charity. There is an old comic song entitled 'I Never Saw a Farmer on a Bike', which ruefully contrasts the wealth of the landowners and subsidised farming community with the rest of the workers. Manufacturers of almost any other product have to find a buyer before they go into big-time production, but under Common Market rules any unsold grain is bought up at a good intervention price which has the effect of keeping the overall price high against world markets. This system positively encourages over-production: quantity at the expense of quality. A familiar story of plenty of artificial fertiliser, weedkiller and insecticides sprayed onto the food we trustingly eat.

Once upon a time, within living memory, local wheat was stone ground at the local mill and taken round for sale by horse and cart. An over seventy-year-old neighbour who told me of his mother buying 14 lb a week and baking wholesome unadulterated bread and cakes for her family, himself led an active outdoor working life and continued part time assisting with vigour for many more years into retirement, as well as maintaining a large garden of fruit and vegetables. He and his contemporary family are also calm, kindly and contented with their lives. It makes one wonder if this good health comes from inherited genes, education and attitudes of the times, or other environmental factors, such as no chemicals, fumes or plastics in the early home, or could it be as straightforward as the more wholesome diet they consumed? Probably a combination of all these factors.

Nowadays wheat tends to be transported all over the country mixed with imported grain, then ground on steel rollers, sifted and refined to remove the larger proportion of its actual goodness before having all sorts of chemicals added to whiten it and improve its keeping qualities. Some is then put into little bags and again carried backwards and forwards all over the country to sell in local shops and supermarkets. The vast bulk is turned into bread, cakes and biscuits ready for us to eat. Here lies one of the greatest causes of trouble, for the bread we still fondly call 'the staff of life' is processed to become the white plastic instigator of all too many illnesses. At present there is still no law which says the additives must be described on the wrapper, so manufacturers let themselves go with bleaches, anti-oxidants, risers, keepers and taste enhancers, to the tune of over twenty additives in some loaves.

Even the seemingly wiser choice of brown bread is not safe as unscrupulous manufacturers often use the same adulterated white dough, just adding malt or a colourant to turn it brown. This fools some customers into thinking they are buying a more wholesome product. You can actually sometimes see the patchy colouration. The description 'wholemeal' means flour or a loaf made from the whole grain. It is preferable to purchase this in a wrapper with the name clearly on it, or from a local baker you have got to know, who will, with luck, tell you exactly what does go into his bread.

A more certain and far more preferable course is to mix and bake your own loaves. Once you have done so, you and the family will be most reluctant to return to shop bread. Ideally, this should be made with wholemeal flour; read the label, it should say something like: 'No additives and nothing taken away'. This means all the bran and germ is still present, so extra bran on cereals etc should not be required. It is a national lunacy that we should pay high prices for bran in little packets, when it has been carefully removed from our flour.

If you prefer a lighter textured and whiter bread, try 81 per cent flour from the health food shop. This should still be free from additives, but has some of the bran removed. The slower-produced, traditionally stone ground flour retains more nutritional elements than mass-produced flour ground at high speed by steel rollers. Beware of white flour with added bran or crushed grains with such comforting titles as 'bran-enriched', or 'granary' flour or bread. If it is proper, unadulterated wholemeal, there is no need for such gimmicks which are designed to attract the new market of health-conscious people.

You will quickly discover that your homemade bread will go stale and even mouldy more readily than shop bread. This is due to the very fact that you are avoiding additives which are put into commercial bread to make it stay fresh and keep longer on the shop shelf. So when you bake, wrap any spare bread well, after it is thoroughly cool, and pop it into the freezer, keeping the current loaf in a box in the fridge. This advice on keeping also applies to the gluten and additive-free recipes which are given in Chapter 7.

It is a good general rule for people who have discovered they are allergic to one or more items to avoid as many additives as possible. They have been found to cause trouble in many cases, as, for example, with a woman who thought it was the gluten in the flour which was upsetting her, only to discover quite accidentally it was one of the additives. She happily returned to eating homemade bread and cakes, using unadulterated flour.

On the debit side of home-baking, one does tend to eat rather more of the delicious homemade produce. More than one gluten allergy has been tracked down – by a sudden increase in the activity of the disease – to the time home-baking with 'strong' flour commenced. Strong flour is imported and has a higher gluten and protein content – these ingredients make bread doughy and able to rise and maintain a nice spongy texture. This is difficult to reproduce in substitute breads. The moral is, if you are fortunate enough not to have an allergy to wheat flours and bread, then do try to ensure you stay that way by sensible eating. That is, do not eat bread or wheat flour at every meal and choose pure wholemeal, so you do not have to resort to added bran. You will not then be risking your health with all kinds of additives, whilst at the same time you will be getting the roughage, germ and minerals naturally present in the grain.

It would also be prudent to avoid as far as possible foods which are obviously over-processed and treated with all sorts of artificial flavourings, dyes, preservatives, taste-enhancers and so on. This applies to sausages, which are mostly a device to use up surplus fat, preserved and cooked meats, ham products in packets and tins, meat and fish pastes, and prepared or packeted desserts, especially items like cheesecake mixes and powders to mix into instant puddings. They all have to have a good helping of preservatives and artificial flavourings in them to make their stale contents taste any good at all. Just like the unadulterated wholemeal bread, they would go mildewed on the grocer's shelf if they were not treated in this way.

For your own and your family's good, try to keep to a diet as near to natural fresh foods as possible. Fresh fruit and vegetables can be prepared in many ways. Once your palate has been re-educated not to expect lots of salt or flavour enhancers, you will really enjoy your food again. Those of us who are lucky enough to have a large garden or allotment can enjoy the additional pleasure of growing some of our own fruit and vegetables and taste them really freshly gathered. Sun-warmed, freshly picked strawberries and tomatoes taste entirely different from those in shops. Also we can eat them with confidence, knowing we have not sprayed them with toxic chemicals a few days before.

The next best is to buy produce from a local nursery or smallholder who genuinely practises organic methods of cultivation, ie uses compost or manure as fertiliser and does not spray with harmful insecticides and herbicides. If you have to purchase from a good greengrocer's shop, as most of us do, then do make sure you wash everything thoroughly in plenty of water.

Recently capturing the notice of the media has been the notion that people who eat a diet high in animal protein are at more risk from all kinds of modern diseases, including cancer. It is no coincidence that the list of safer foods I have suggested you try out, in order to alleviate the pain of rheumatoid arthritis, eliminates all the modern farmed animal protein products, ie meats, animal fats, milk, cheeses, creams, poultry and even eggs. Contrary to popular folk-belief, these can be safely as well as adequately replaced with vegetable protein in the form of nuts and pulses, beans and peas of all sorts and textured soya products, together with fresh fish.

The majority of sea fish is the only living protein which is still truly allowed to grow in its wild environment, where it eats a naturally evolved diet and gets plenty of exercise to thin and refine the muscles which we eventually eat. By the same token, some fish farming can be a sad development for healthy nutrition, so when shopping, beware the tempting treat of the now cheaper priced salmon and trout which have been reared crowded in ponds or cages, where they are denied a normal life and exercise.

Because my illness had gone on so long unchecked and I was

eating foods which were harming me all that time quite unknowingly, the poisons built up in my body and I found I was unfortunately unable to eat quite a large number of everyday foods. At first it seemed rather worrying in case there was not sufficient left to supply proper nourishment and, equally important, enjoyment in eating.

After nine years of feeling better and better, I am glad to be able to report that an almost vegan diet has no drawbacks at all healthwise if you are sensible about it and eat plenty of variety of what is left, spending the money saved at the butcher and the dairy on more exotic and interesting fruits and vegetables. I can still eat most fish, and a little white meat – chicken or turkey – for a treat, but even here I find if I have a large helping, or a food too often repeated on the menu I begin to feel decidedly sluggish and out of sorts for anything between a couple of hours and several days.

I am really suggesting that more of us revert to the wholefood, more vegetarian diet of our hunter-gatherer and early farming forebears. There are still countless examples of this in the world today, where a balanced diet continues to maintain a healthy population of millions with a healthy eco-system for the land on which we all ultimately depend. Some of the rice-growing areas in mountainous terrain with neat, terraced fields for irrigation, and with glacial melt-water rich in minerals to fertilise the crop, continue to produce health-giving food after thousands of years of careful gardening with the only addition being the return of organic waste.

In South America, the layered system, in which maize (which we call sweetcorn) shelters beans of various sorts around its stems with squash as a ground-covering vegetable, supplies the indigenous people with starch, protein and vegetables to provide a nutritious, balanced mix of tasty wholefood with perhaps the occasional variant of a treat of animal milk and meat from goats, pigs and chickens, economically grazing the more inaccessible corners of their world. This successful eco-system, evolved over many generations, also keeps the land fertile, with the beans able to use nitrogen from the air to nourish the soil, plants and in turn man, whilst the farmers wisely compost and return all organic matter to be recycled once more.

Another useful habit which can be advantageously copied from Eastern countries is to sprout beans and seeds in jars in your own kitchen and then enjoy them raw in salads of all kinds. This practice increases the nutritional value of the dried seeds and because they are not cooked, nothing is destroyed. It is wise practice to enjoy at least one meal a day of completely raw chopped vegetables. Many kinds of refreshing salads can be prepared with a simple but effective variety of dressings. Raw cabbage in coleslaw has a taste all of its own and can be varied with different additions. This way none of the elusive vitamins are lost and your health and vitality will improve. If going on a journey, or simply each day to school or work, a small plastic container per person of mixed layered salad keeps and travels well and is more refreshing than sandwiches. It can be topped with shrimps, tuna or salmon, but as these products do not keep well once opened, it may be better to carry a small tin and a tin-opener to open it just before eating. It is simple to eat this meal with a plastic fork and saves all that wondering which of the restaurant foods would do you the least harm.

– 12 –

Environmental Causes Of Allergies

Until now I have emphasised the need to trace and eliminate your staple food allergies as described in Chapter 6 and have hardly mentioned all the other adverse environmental factors. This is because arthritics seem to be more affected by the food they eat than anything else. However, there are some people whose arthritis is severely aggravated, if not caused, by other environmental factors.

Amongst these factors are the dreadful hazards of various types of toxic dusts at workplaces, the dangers of which are at last very gradually being recognised. Men who toil down coalmines, or quarry for slate, spend years of their life breathing in fine dust particles which accumulate in the delicate tissues of their lungs. This can gradually reduce the usable area until breathlessness and chronic ill-health become the norm. Then there is the even more insidious poisoning from asbestos dust, which can cause illness years after workers have left the polluted environment. Asbestos causes not simply a clogging of the lungs but a disease which can take many forms, and it can be very difficult for the worker to link it directly with his disease when it comes to claiming compensation. These hazards were known about for years before any real effort was made to protect the lives of the people working with them. It seems a sad reflection on our society that it is only pressure from masses of people, if they are fortunate to have a story interesting enough for the media, that may eventually bring about reform in health aspects of this sort. More modern hazards range from diesel oils and weedkillers to radiation.

Then there exist the more hidden dangers of alien fumes breathed in at the workplace, be it a factory with heavy industrial processes, or a workshop with glues, resin and plastic processes, a print works or whatever.

Modern buildings are often centrally heated at far too high a temperature for good health. Shops, offices, hotels and even hospitals are so warm that the inmates have to discard many layers of outdoor clothes to be able to tolerate the atmosphere. Unfortunate short-term visitors and shoppers dressed in clothes sensible for the streets have to suffer in silence for the duration of their visit – which is often curtailed simply by the desire to breathe fresh air and cool down again.

In order to maintain this high temperature the warm air is recirculated time and again by air-conditioning plants. It is passed through filters and then the excess dryness is partly overcome by humidifiers spraying tiny droplets of moisture into the warm air before being used again.

These tanks of warm stagnant water are excellent breeding ground for many types of bacteria, which are then spread throughout the building causing mysterious allergic reactions amongst staff who happen to be sensitive, from sore eyes and throats, coughs and colds to Legionnaire's disease, which was first identified as responsible for killing many people amongst a convention of American 'legionnaires' in a Philadelphia hotel and has since been responsible for deaths in Britain. Some of those infected did not even enter the contaminated buildings but simply breathed in the fumes as they walked past and had the extractor fan waft the stale, bacteria-charged air their way.

How much better for health and economy it would be if as well as regularly sterilising the humidifying tanks, these buildings were only heated to a tolerable background heat with the occupants wearing extra clothes, as we all did in our homes until recent years.

It is not only the people who work in these buildings or factories who are at risk. In order better to protect them, large extractors are fitted which channel the industrial dust and fumes to the outer air, often only at rooftop level, sometimes guided into a tall chimney in the hopes of dilution in the upper atmosphere. Diluted they may be, but all these released gases and dusts have to find a home somewhere. Much of the pollution stays around the towns and cities where it was discharged. Some can be detected by smell, some not, but we have no option but to breathe it all in. With our prevailing westerly airstream, part of our industrial waste and gases which reaches higher altitudes is conveniently carried away from our own area only to fall, it is now acknowledged, as polluted acid rain over the less industrialised areas of our neighbours, denuding their forests and laying waste the life in their once abundant rivers and lakes.

There is not much we can do as individuals to rectify these historical wrongs, apart from joining ecology-minded groups who exert pressure on the government to take more heed of the needs of the planet as a whole rather than desecrate the whole earth for the short-term advantage of a few.

Yet there is a lot we can do to improve the atmosphere of our home and workplace. It is well worth doing because people who are allergic, and that is what you are if you have now found some food substances have been making you ill, do tend to be sensitive to more than one factor at a time. For instance, one woman became ill after having a new kitchen fitted. It was eventually discovered that the varnish finish on the wooden doors of the expensive cupboard units were exuding fumes which upset her. The solution was to strip off the synthetic varnish and use a more old-fashioned one which was carefully tested on the cook before application to the doors!

If your symptoms become worse, it is well worth looking around for a change in your circumstances that coincided with your deterioration. Let us hope it is not as drastic and expensive as the kitchen units story, but petrochemical based paints and plastics do have a habit of triggering reactions in sensitive people, so it would be prudent to carry out a fume test before painting your room. Just as you can conduct the pulse test with sample foods, sit down in an airy place and note your pulse rate and how you feel. Then open the paint can and cautiously smell the contents. Close it again, take your pulse and note any dizziness, nausea, etc. If your pulse rate is raised and you react adversely to the fumes, just imagine what it will be like living in a room with them permeating from the walls over a considerable time. Better to try a different type of paint.

This test can be used for all the chemicals used in the home. You don't think you use many? Well, take a look in your kitchen, bathroom and cleaning cupboards. All those aerosol sprays should be suspect, for a start. Highly perfumed polishes, cleaners, oven cleaners, air fresheners, deodorants and hairsprays also contain propellants to which many people have adverse reactions, not only people with arthritis. After these, test your range of detergents from washing powder to washing up liquid and choose milder, more naturally based ones if possible. Detergents should be well-rinsed off china and cutlery as they can be harmful to eat. You will also be doing your local river or sea, or wherever your drains end up, a favour if you use less detergent!

Now, what about your bottle of bleach and lavatory cleaner, and spirit to clean stains? The list of such things is usually pretty long. All these, which can be breathed into the lungs, should be handled with proper caution and you should use them as little as possible to avoid absorbing their fumes. Garden pest control chemicals naturally should be avoided, as well as fly-spray in the home, including the solid type recommended for lofts and cupboards.

Other invisible components of the air we have no option but to breathe are the spores of various fungi and moulds. These are present everywhere of course, but in the less disturbed air of rooms housing substances on which they can grow easily, you could be experiencing a more concentrated dose. It is worth checking the backs of cupboards and odd corners for leather goods, which grow moulds to perfection, and keep food areas clean. Paint into corners and behind pipes to assure nothing is lodged and forgotten, moulding away happily. Good ventilation will also help disperse moulds in the air and keep the rooms drier.

The rotting vegetation in the soil is essential for plant life regeneration, but the moulds produced can have a detrimental effect on a small proportion of people living with pot plants in the house. People with chest conditions could advantageously have a trial period with pot-plants banished. If this trial period brings about an improvement in health, the plants could be tried repotted in sterilised soil, or sprayed to kill off any existing moulds before readmitting them to the home. Do the spraying outside and allow to disperse well before bringing them inside again.

A considerable number of people, particularly those with multiple allergies, only have to enter a gas-heated room to feel dizzy and ill. It is not the heat, but the fumes of the only partly burnt gas which does it. If you have lived in a gas-polluted atmosphere for years you may not realise it is the gas which is causing you to be unwell. Naturally, your own reactions may be different ones, as the susceptible area of each allergic person varies and it is this diversity which can make allergies so tricky to recognise and treat. Typical symptoms, however, are a raised pulse rate, day-long fatigue with loss of vitality, and almost any other symptoms of ill health: nausea, headache, indigestion, and so on.

To compound the difficulties of tracking down an allergy to gas is the leakage problem. It might not be enough to turn off the gas boiler and the cooker and use an electric ring for a while. Gas can enter our homes in considerable volume, as gas pipes can be up to a hundred years old. All joints are vulnerable to deterioration with age, vibration or fatigue, so it is by no means exceptional to find small gas leaks in homes. These might invade the house with a dose too diluted to explode or smell strongly of gas, but quite sufficient to make a person living there feel off-colour, if not downright ill. The

Gas Board will test your pipes and installation for leakage if you suspect this may be the case. The service is free for the first thirty minutes of inspection, but you have to pay for any repairs necessary.

If you feel it might be a good idea to test your own or your family's susceptibility to gas fumes, I can only suggest you plan this year's holiday at an all-electric establishment in a country area, where other fumes are hopefully going to be low too. Be sure to choose a holiday home with no gas pipes entering the establishment.

One of the other sources of fumes you are likely to encounter on such a holiday, however, are those emitted by traffic. Travel sickness is greatly worsened by exhaust fumes getting into the body of the car, so some people find they become ill in some vehicles and not others. A good deal of travel sickness is caused not by motion, but by the fumes. Some countries have a far lower amount of pollution allowed in exhaust gases than here in the UK and it is up to us to continue to press for this. The lead content of petrol is quite a separate issue and, of course, this could be beneficially reduced if the politics of big business were to allow this. Meanwhile, infants continue to be pushed in prams or walked along pavements at vehicle-exhaust height where, as the most susceptible members of the public, they are treated to the greatest exposure.

If, on taking a holiday or exchanging homes with a friend or relative away from gas and exhaust fumes, you or members of your family feel markedly better, then it is well worth considering having the mains gas cut off outside your home and changing to other means of heating and cooking. Or, as I advised a person who had the misfortune to suffer due to having a smoke-testing station for firemen set up next door, move house.

Another risk to avoid is putting into our food traces of aluminium from cooking pans. Every housewife knows that cooking fruit in an aluminium pan leaves it clean and shiny because the acid reacts to dissolve away a thin layer of the metal. Where else can it go but into the food? Aluminium is a soft metal and traces of it can be worn away when stirring with steel utensils during cooking. Even enamelled ironware is not safe because the cheaper makes leach out lead and cadmium metals from their glazes. The best material I have heard recommended to date is stainless steel which, although expensive, should last a lifetime of careful use and not contribute to your inner pollution. Iron pots are thought to be safe, but are heavy to handle.

The next source of air pollution worth a mention here is the entirely self-induced one of tobacco smoke. Not always avoidable if you are breathing this in secondhand from friends and relations, this is a very real cause of nicotine tar pollution in the home and public places. In these more enlightened times the trend is towards segregating smokers in public places, but there is always a minority of inconsiderate people quite prepared to light up in smoke-free places. A coach trip can be ruined when although sitting near the front where 'No Smoking' signs are displayed, another passenger insists on smoking, and the fumes can make a sensitive person feel travel-sick. I appreciate that those folk who became hooked on tobacco before the dangers of it were publicised have their own problems in trying to give it up, but this is a subject well covered by others.

Arthritic people, along with many other sufferers from different allergic conditions, are also sensitive to extremes in temperature. They cannot happily tolerate a very cold temperature, nor one that is too warm for them. I often joke that my thermostat has gone wrong, although I am becoming slightly better in this respect. On balance if I cannot have the happy medium of spring or autumn all year round, I prefer cold weather as I can wrap up warmly and still get on, but on those rare hot summer days I wilt and cannot summon up the energy to do much at all – at least not nearly as much as I wish to.

There is a lot of folklore about damp conditions causing rheumatism. I have come to the conclusion this is because the cold and damp make existing aches and pains feel worse, rather than being the cause of them. Warm, dry housing conditions certainly help to make one feel better. When I was first diagnosed as having arthritis I was living in an area of clay soils beside the sea. It was seriously recommended that we should move to an area such as Brighton, where the chalk subsoil allowed freer drainage and thus a drier atmosphere! Because of family circumstances, this was not possible and in fact I now live in a marshy area where the mist often lies over the fields and water in the early evening and morning, giving spectacular sunrises and sunsets, but having no detectable effect on my aches and pains.

Well-aired clothes and bedding – also highly recommended for arthritics – cannot always be provided on some of the sailing expeditions I have been on. Once again, spending all day in sea or rain-soaked clothes and night in damp sleeping bags, although uncomfortable, has no effect on my joints as long as I have been able to keep relatively warm in windproof outer garments and have been able to keep to the diet which suits me. Inactivity and the wrong foods are my worst enemies.

Proof seems to be provided every day that the illnesses of old age are not so inevitable as we thought. The so-called degenerative diseases of Western society are being linked to incorrect eating habits. Senility, difficulty of movement, incontinence and personality diminishment are all features of old age which have been helped by elimination diets whereas in the past it has been suggested that only those people with a strong will have retained their faculties into old age.

– 13 –

The Need For Specialist Help

The body is a wonderfully complex machine, and has a highly involved chemical factory. All our actions, from digesting and utilising food as fuel, to running, walking, sleeping, thinking and reasoning, feeling and growing, are chemical reactions of one kind or another. No wonder the vital fuel in the form of food and drink which we inject into this microcosm of a factory is so important. If we were to purposely take a known poison such as arsenic, we would expect things to go wrong, yet we cheerfully consume all sorts of other dubious chemicals in the form of drugs or hidden in prepared, convenience and adulterated foods, and expect our bodies to cope without complaint.

Complementary, fringe or alternative medicine covers many different aspects of health and treatments. It includes qualified acupuncturists, osteopaths, herbalists, faith healers, masseurs and so on, who usually have to make a reasonable charge in order to live whilst practising their skills to the benefit of their fellows.

Unfortunately, there are a few people with less altruistic aims who produce convincing-sounding equipment, treatments, gadgets, and so on which turn out to be mere gimmicks. The medical profession, on the other hand, as a monitored body, is in a good position to help those with allergies, if only it could and would. I would like to see dietary control used as an official weapon against the common enemy of pain. Is it too much to ask that we should have official specialists in dietary control as well as in the many other fields now available at modern hospitals?

There is a different school of thought which is demonstrated in the following contribution from an equally concerned person, Erick James, who feels that it will take far too long for the medical profession to be additionally trained and to accept this new method. He therefore sees the need for a separate body of 'allergy specialists' treating people in a private, consultative, but professional way. There seems no way of judging which would be most helpful, but I feel both should be considered.

Mr James says: 'Unsuspectingly allergic people can in effect continue to mildly poison themselves each day and this can often ultimately cause a cumulative build-up their body cannot cope with any longer. Eventually some interior part will partly or wholly break down, resulting in one or more of sixty illnesses which it is suspected are caused needlessly by allergies.

The drugs that doctors prescribe can rarely do more than partly suppress the pain and misery involved because they cannot get to the root cause of the victim's problem. If the illness is caused because the person is allergic, then the only way to remove the problem is for the person to determine which element of their daily food or environment happens to be antagonistic to their interior bodily functions. It may be a minor or a fixed allergen which they can cease eating or drinking or replace with an alternative food which is inoffensive to their system. It could be that this alternative is not so tasty as the forbidden fruit, at least at first, but that is a price you pay for regaining better health.

The present breakdown is in getting the need for this simple sort of do-it-yourself treatment across to the sufferer. One major way for a few at present, if they are still active enough, is to go to a large public library and look in one of the very few books that have been published that discuss arthritis as an allergic disease. Doctors' waiting rooms and hospitals would have fewer patients if sufferers from allergies had already diagnosed and successfully treated themselves.

There is little chance of a family doctor or orthodox hospital saying to a patient, 'You do not need an X-ray or operation for your illness, and any drugs we could give you for it will only lessen the pain for a while, because we think the cause is that you may be allergic to something or other. Consequently, it would be best if you study the books on the subject.'

Alas, the workaday medical world of doctors, specialists or even the nursing profession does not operate like that. Instead, there is a closed shop where it is difficult for any outsider to contribute or assist with real patient-caring for the sick.

Allergists are the first to agree that food allergy, intolerance or aversion may not be the prime cause of many illnesses. Allergist practitioners insist that the chronically ill patient must be separated from the acutely ill, and no alternative medicine will take its place if an operation is necessary. What clinical allergists say is that if a person is making themselves ill, however unwittingly, as a result of being allergic to something, then before ever it becomes serious enough to need an operation, the patient should be given every opportunity and encouragement to first ascertain if they have an allergy and, if so, to remove its influence to see whether the body then heals itself. If that happens, they will almost certainly never reach the stage where a serious operation becomes necessary.

There is no conventional medical treatment in the world one fraction as effective as your own body in its capacity to heal itself, provided it is given half a chance. If you happen, as Pat Byrivers was, to be unknowingly allergic to milk and wheat, then you will only get worse if you persist in eating these particular foodstuffs, for the simple reason that your body cannot go on tolerating them and is making you ill as if to prove it.

Recently, on behalf of the Help Yourself to Less Pain Society, I wrote in the *Journal of Alternative Medicine* an article called 'Allergies: A Field For Non-Medical Specialists', recording that in 1984 there had been a couple of television programmes about allergies which, if accurately done, could be a step in the right direction.

A *World In Action* programme showed that despite specialist evidence already proving that some diseases could be corrected by discontinuing certain foods, the rest of the medical profession would not listen.

We feel that the average general practitioner already takes on too large a range of treatments and drug alleviation and that in the separate field of allergies there should be non-medical specialists.

Such clinical technicians do not have to be qualified doctors, because they should issue absolutely no drugs of any sort. Neither have they any cause to carry out any surgery, or make anything more than superficial examination of already exposed areas like the face and hands in cases such as eczema.

As allergists, we submit that a considerable proportion of those in doctors' waiting-rooms and in hospitals are there because they are allergic. They are unnecessarily ill simply because, without their realising it, they are regularly eating something which does not agree with them. The offending substance could be oranges, onions, hamburgers, coffee, chocolate, sausages, or any of the scores of other consumables we regularly eat.

As specialist allergists we feel we should be encouraged, for the wellbeing of needless sufferers, to spread our harmless communications. If the home tests we prescribe are seriously followed by the patient with or without the consent of their doctor, and without or with their drugs, only good will result.

If, after adequate tests, the sufferer feels no better or cannot trace having an allergy, or other intolerance, then no harm will have been done and we will recommend the person involved to consider other complementary and holistic medicines as might seem best fitted to their particular case: homoeopathy, acupuncture, clinical hypnosis, osteopathy, natural therapeutic and physical therapy, relaxation, remedial massage, vegetarianism, or even aerobics or gentle jogging if the person is fit enough.'

– 14 –

Taking Responsibility For Your Own Life

The Chinese have a sensible system of paying their health advisors. A physician is engaged to keep the client in good health with a natural balance of herbs and dietary advice. While this is successful they pay him a fee. When the advisor fails and the patient becomes ill, payment is discontinued until the physician has managed to heal them, when presumably they are back at work so can afford to pay once more for their continued good health. The logic of this method is very attractive, with the patient paying while in a position to earn and the physician having an incentive to maintain the health of his clients.

In the Western world most of us wait until we are feeling decidedly ill, or very inconvenienced, worried or embarrassed by our symptoms before we can be persuaded to get professional assistance. Sometimes it is tragically too late for any remedial action. In other instances the task of healing is made more difficult, drastic and prolonged because the illness has had the opportunity to cause havoc in one direction or another. On the other hand we are actively discouraged from going along to the doctor with every trivial ache and pain because they are inundated with work.

By historical accident Western medicine has come to place far more emphasis on alleviation than on prevention of illness. It is an entirely laudable motive to sincerely wish to make better a person who is ill. When a person goes to his doctor in distress and pain we are fortunate in having a health service staffed in the main by conscientious and skilled people. Regrettably, I tend to feel it is the system which may not be helping us attain the better state of health envisaged at the instigation of this centrally funded health service, supported by individual contributions.

Very recently there has been a slight move by the media and government towards health education in such areas as tobacco smoking and too much fatty food in the diet. This has happened after years of effort by researchers, and only after thousands of people have met with an untimely death as a result of these two bad habits. It is still not made generally known that lung cancer is not the only serious illness caused by smoking, nor heart attacks the only possible result of too much high fat food.

Preventative health care, once established in conjunction with the cure-them-afterwards approach, ought to be a cost-effective policy early on in the regime. Naturally I am mainly interested in allergy detection and the prevention of illness through these means. I am sure the cost of a small, chemically clean ward, with staff trained in elimination diet techniques, is less than the high technology of X-ray machines, operating theatres, and so on. To the patient the difference in treatment would be much appreciated when they realised the pain and trauma they could be avoiding by adopting a slightly different lifestyle and eating habits early on. We may not yet understand fully how it works but it undeniably does have a high success rate amongst those who try it for themselves here in the UK as well as the much higher percentage of the population in the USA who utilise the dietary approach.

As in so many other fashions, we seem to follow a lead set by the more progressive Americans when it comes to health consciousness. This may be because they do not have a high standard of free health care and so cannot afford to be ill, in spite of the fact that everyone who can possibly do so contributes to expensive private health insurance schemes. In other words most people have taken responsibility for their own wellbeing and are thus vitally interested in the effects of exercise and healthy eating on both their figure and their health in general. We may be slightly amused, if not superior, about the craze for this or that health fad in California, but the incidence of heart disease in the USA is now far lower than that in the UK and it is still falling. Who knows what the statistics for other degenerative diseases may show? The population in general certainly seem to have a more energetic attitude to their work and play. Staple food allergies are far more accepted as part of the self-help health pattern and the cytotoxic test previously described has been used by many well-known actors and athletes, with positive results in the improvement of health and vitality.

It is easy to understand the attraction of complex apparatus to the medics, scientists and technicians involved. Wonderful body scanners and optic probes, lasers and so on are great feats of engineering skill and impart even more mystique and reflected glory upon the particular departments involved. They also make great slogans for charities to use to collect money from the public.

In contrast the more homespun and simple techniques advocated in this book may not have a similar instant appeal to the imagination, but an examination of the cost effectiveness of this method should endear itself to the heart of any budget-minded politician.

Take an example with which I am only too familiar. A child of say 14 years suddenly shows all the signs of rheumatoid arthritis. Many tests are carried out to confirm that this is indeed the case. As the disease progresses, X-rays confirm the deterioration of joints and specialists' consultations and costs mount up, together with the inevitable endless repeat prescriptions for expensive drugs. Outpatient treatment several times a week, punctuated with hospitalisation for intensive therapy now and again, culminates in operations to relieve or replace the worst joints. Quite an expensive scenario over the entire lifetime of the unlucky victim, but to this has been added the cost to the State of sickness and other benefits for a person eventually unable to work at all.

Now substitute a month in a special unit to isolate the chemical or foods which are triggering off these original symptoms, followed up by occasional specialist guidance by an allergist, and care at a community health centre. The child should be back at school quite soon, with every prospect of following his or her chosen career as long as he or she follows the new regime. If the patient runs into difficulties with this, sympathetic after-care consultations should be available. There would be no expensive technology, no drugs, no pension, no nursing.

To put it all into such crude money terms may offend, but financial considerations do seem to carry more weight than the huge saving in human suffering implicit in the above example.

Suffering of this sort is impossible to describe accurately. It is said that a doctor who has been ill himself is the best one to go to, as he will understand your problems better. I must agree that when I got a dose of shingles affecting my head, eye and ear my GP, who had just recovered from the same complaint, was most understanding about my miseries! Most healthy people have no possible way of knowing what it is like to have a really bad, long-term illness. If the victims complain they are gradually shunned as a 'misery' or a 'bore'. If they do not mention the pain they may be admired as stoical, or more likely accepted as ill, but not really suffering.

Closer questioning of many of these patients, as I have done, reveals a different story. They are usually in considerable pain most of the time and, contrary to what some people believe, you do not get used or inured to this state. It simply wears you out. To combat the pain and inflammation the patients are put on powerful drugs which dull the mind and frequently have detrimental side effects, some of which are more serious than others, but all of which have an adverse effect on the patient as a person.

I am the first to admit I have been extremely lucky in that steroids have suited me reasonably well, producing side effects which are certainly bad enough, but not as serious as for some people – at least so far. Several times my medical advisors have tried to take me off them altogether. Each attempt has ended in an increased dosage for a while to get me back to a manageable norm. The withdrawal symptoms in my case consist of headaches (which I very rarely experience at any other time), depression to the extent of constant crying, and of course a violent return of the pain, inflammation and swelling which nothing else seems to relieve. Knowing the alternatives, I persevere with very gradual reduction, but even one less tablet a week in a total of seventeen culminates in a lot more pain with loss of good spirits. The moral is not to reach a state where one has to take drugs in the first place, but all those years ago I did not know the consequences nor have any alternative.

In the light of my dramatic improvement in health since I discovered how to eliminate my allergens, I seriously feel that, had this dietary approach been tried early on in my illness, there would have been no need for me to start to take steroids at all.

At the time I first discovered my allergens, I was feeling really ill with increasing pain and stiffness in spite of a gradual increase in steroids. As soon as I ceased to eat all the wrong (for me) foods, my pain diminished rapidly and I was initially able to reduce the dosage. But the problem is that if one takes artificial cortisone for a number of years the body practically ceases to manufacture its own natural supply. After nearly thirty years on these drugs mine has apparently forgotten how to do this and so I am stuck with taking steroids for the foreseeable future.

Rheumatoid arthritis is such an all-pervasive and powerful illness that if it is going to be treated by a drug it seems to require a powerful one to combat it. Any drug taken into the delicate balance of the human body will affect every tissue in some way, so whilst any given medication might help the pain and inflammation, its residual effects can be multiple and may in time be worse than the original pain. Now and again one hears reports in the press and media of a drug being withdrawn because it is dangerous. The many hundreds of human stories of pain and distress are not reported – just the statistics of alarming side-effects and reactions which cannot be explained away. The investment into research and production of such drugs is so huge nowadays that the profit to be made seems to be more important than the cure they set out to find. Sometimes scandals are investigated and occasionally reported to the general public. The specific pills are withdrawn, the huge drug firms cut their losses and redouble their efforts to find yet another so-called wonder drug. You, the patient, with the very real problem of constant pain and disability, are the target of all this industrial intrigue. Your money and that of millions like you is the potential profit being sought.

It is human nature to hope for miracles and in the field of arthritis the most obvious miracle to look for is a wonder cure produced by some expert from afar. Twenty-five years ago a well-intentioned doctor tried to cheer me up, after saying there was nothing else he could do, by remarking on the research being carried out by drug companies. He said that I was so young that something was bound to come up that would help me before I was too crippled. But the more I read of deaths, loss of bone marrow, loss of sight, inability to go out in the sunshine due to skin sensitivity, wrecked digestive systems and so on, the more I come to feel we are looking in the wrong direction for our miracle.

Therefore I most earnestly suggest that if you are starting to suffer from a few aches and pains and your doctor proposes a course of anti-inflammatory drugs, you question him about any known side effects before accepting them and at the same time check your eating habits with the lists in Chapter 6. I do not want to be unduly pessimistic, but a few aches and pains sometimes have a nasty habit of persisting and worsening before you know where you are.

If, as is more than likely to be the case with serious readers of this book, you have already reached the stage of too much pain and are taking some form of medication, then I trust you are sufficiently convinced to start a really searching analysis of your staple foods.

When you are feeling the benefit of this, it is time to go along to your doctor and ask him if he feels it would be safe for you gradually to reduce the number of tablets you are taking. If you know for certain which are simply painkillers and feel you can manage with less, by all means gradually reduce these yourself, but for all other drugs professional advice is a must. It is entirely up to you and the doctor concerned whether you feel your relationship will bear discussing diet or environment as a factor in your improvement, but that is not essential. Just explain you are feeling a little better and would prefer to take less drugs if possible. You will be amazed and grateful at the way the myriad of little inconveniences you have been putting up with as unavoidable can start to disappear.

I mentioned earlier the difficulty of communication with your medical advisors when you are feeling very ill. The typical British stiff upper lip reflex reaction when someone asks 'How are you?' is to politely reply, 'Very well, thank you', even when friends meet in the doctor's waiting room when it is obvious they would not be there if this were really the case. But when your doctor asks how you are, make a special effort to describe how you really feel; he is not a thought reader and cannot help you unless he understands the full extent of the problem. By this, I do not mean you should ramble on about how poorly you feel, but assemble your facts before you go and describe them as shortly and accurately as possible.

In return, let us hope your doctor will communicate more fully and honestly with you than is all too frequently the case at the moment. Perhaps doctors are advised to add to their air of mystery by not telling the patient every last detail they happen to know about the particular illness in question. Nothing must be done to spoil the implicit trust most patients have in their doctors, so how can the GP admit that very little is known about, or can be done about disease 'X', except that with rest and luck nature will take its course and you will feel better?

Then there is the theory that the patient would not

understand the medical details or would worry unduly if these were given. On the first score it is up to the doctor to simplify and explain things so that the patient and his close relatives do understand something of what is happening. Secondly, fear of an unknown outcome is usually very much worse in the imaginings of an unwell person and his concerned family than knowing the truth.

It comes down to a basic human right to have the information which affects that person more than any other. Patients need to know in order to be able to co-operate in the treatment of their illness and to help establish a positive attitude towards it. To hide the truth from a patient is one of the most unkind things that can be done. What is a person to think if, after all sorts of tests, they are reassured it is nothing serious? Unless they rapidly recover, they still have the problem, but with no hope of any improvement and the feeling that nobody understands how they feel. If relatives connive at this deception, one conclusion the patient could draw is that they do not care that he is feeling so ill: after all, his thinking and reasoning ability is not at its best at such times. It is not a good idea for a parent or spouse always to hide their real feelings and put on a bright, brave face in front of the patient. For heaven's sake let your emotions show occasionally, even to the extent of having a good cry together; you can then start to rebuild your lives from a better basis of trust and mutual understanding.

Take for example a child with arthritis for whom it became necessary to have major hip surgery. The mother was told this would be very painful – especially the manipulative therapy directly after the operation. She was advised to stay away during these times. This loving mother could be seen weeping in the corridors, but managed never to break down in front of her child, who always saw her smiling as though everything were normal and correct. True communication of their mutual fears and feelings could not help but be impaired.

In the UK at the moment it is almost universal policy that the notes on any patient be a closely guarded secret. This is fine, if they are being kept confidential from prying eyes, but please not from the person most concerned – the patient. For some reason, as soon as anyone admits to being unwell and becomes that unit to be called 'the patient' they suddenly find their intellectual status takes a nose-dive. Why must the temporarily unwell be treated as imbeciles and hardly consulted when it is they who know more about how they feel than anyone else? From the moment the sufferer is admitted into hospital and deprived of his clothes, he is treated very kindly, but at best as some sort of erring child. Consultants and retinue whisper annoyingly out of earshot, all and sundry, from the newest little trainee nurse upwards, seem able to read the notes but not the patient who is most affected by the doctors' decisions. Patients are the last to hear how they are progressing and what to expect as they come out of an anaesthetic, or recuperate from stroke, heart attack or operation, except by comparing notes with other patients, which can be very unsatisfactory and alarming. The patient rarely sees his X-rays or other test results, nor are they explained to him.

Too many patients do not understand what the drugs they are taking are supposed to do, let alone that they should watch out for any side effects. Some doctors feel that if they tell their patient he may feel dizzy or sick on such and such a medication, the patient will thus be dizzy and sick by the power of suggestion. Maybe some would, but it might be safer if patients were warned to stop taking them under certain circumstances.

I would like to see everybody work towards a more open medical system with better communication on both sides. We have suffered long enough the 'them and us' attitude of our present regime. By and large many people are far more intelligent and willing to listen than they are given credit for and it is up to the establishment to break down some of the barriers in order to obtain fuller communication and co-operation with their patients. The art of communication could be included in the curriculum so the person responsible, or nurse concerned, tells the patient the basics of their position and is willing to answer questions truthfully.

It was suggested to me by a specialist whom I had consulted when at a very low ebb that my arthritis was mainly in my imagination and all the visible symptoms were caused by a wish for attention. This sort of talk can be extremely distressing for the stricken patient, when the very last thing they want to wish upon themselves is the severe pain and misery they are experienching. All of the relatively small number of sufferers I have had the opportunity to discuss this with have an extremely well motivated desire to feel better, not only for their own benefit, but to avoid being a nuisance or a burden upon the very people from whom this medical specialist suggested they were seeking attention.

Amongst people with minor joint disorders there may well be a few who exaggerate their troubles, but amongst the seriously ill to whom my remarks are mainly addressed, there is no need to add psychosomatic pains – they are fully occupied with the very real ones existing already. By this I do not dismiss the useful contribution of positive thinking. It is amazing the difference a surprise visitor or the prospect of an enjoyable outing can make to the way one feels on any particular day. It is all too easy to get into a rut of just trickling along at a comfortable pace and not extending yourself with seemingly unnecessary extra activity. If every day becomes the same, it is difficult to motivate yourself into doing even all that you should about the house.

If you have to get up early to get the house spick and span and prepare meals for visitors, it is surprising how much more you get done and how much better you feel. So do not hesitate to undertake a few extra chores as you begin to feel better, preferably activities which take you outside the home and your usual tasks. Visit an elderly or lonely neighbour for a cheerful chat, taking a homemade cake or perhaps offer to do some shopping; babysit for youngsters, volunteer to assist the Red Cross or local hospital. These are small tasks but ones which will make a positive contribution to others, yet at the same time extend you and give immense personal satisfaction.

Now you are feeling so much better and getting out and about, it is time to give a little more attention to your appearance. How long is it since you changed your hairstyle? Does your present one really suit the new, vibrant you? If, like me, you still have difficulty reaching your hair, why not forget about curls with all the problems of perms and curlers and get your hairdresser to style you a modern, less fussy look which allows your hair to shine and take a more natural line and is relatively trouble-free? Are you sure your make-up still suits you and do you need as much? Why not get the younger element to help you take stock, without going in for anything too different? What about your clothes? Have you become a little bit conservative from having to choose items which are easy to get into and fasten in the front? Try some more carefree, casual clothes.

I know clothes can be very expensive nowadays and I have my own solution. Whenever I see a bargain I try to afford it there and then. In fact I have made a bit of an entertaining hobby in seeing how little I can pay for clothes I like. Look at market stalls and sales racks. The most unpromising places can come up with all sorts of treasures. I have a pair of slacks which cost only a pound in a London store; they were brand new and perfect in all respects – they even drip dry, and don't need to be ironed! Similar ones seen elsewhere were twelve times the price so they were a wonderful bargain. I recently bought several British-made long-sleeved, roll-neck jumpers at fifty pence each. On a market stall, all heaped together, they looked like junk, but individually examined and away from the market atmosphere, friends cannot believe the price and quality. Of course, you do not have to tell your friends of your astuteness, but I generally cannot resist doing so, or sometimes rewarding their kindness with one of my bargain buys.

Of course, if having arthritis has not meant you have suffered financially, this approach may not appeal to you, but everyone loves a bargain and the pleasure of the chase pursued at odd moments: it makes shopping much more fun. But be warned – it is not worth buying something simply because it is cheap. Make sure it is perfect, fits and suits you before you take the plunge. Whatever else, it adds a little spice to ordinary living.

I give this aside into one of my harmless pleasures as an example of turning what could be a problem into a fun activity. Another way of turning each day into positive enjoyment rather than a chore or a duty, is to structure or plan in advance. But do not be too set in your ways so you are able to change in mid-course if an opportunity for something else occurs. It all helps in your battle against pain and despondency and I am sure if necessary you can think of many other examples. If you can wake up each day and think of several pleasurable things you are going to do, it encourages you to get up and get going, even if the tasks set are not all fun in the accepted sense. Just small achievements in your private world, such as reorganising a cupboard, painting a wall or a picture, making some curtains, taking your first bus or coach ride for years – the possibilities are endless. There is a lot to be said for the well-worn advice of joining an adult education class and learning something new, whilst at the same time meeting some different people. Have you ever fancied dressmaking, pottery, watercolours, a new language ...? If you happen to possess a special skill, have you ever thought of passing it on at such classes, or volunteering to teach at an adult literacy or numeracy centre? Some of these classes are held in the daytime now.

If you can say 'thank-you' for another fulfilled day before you drop off to sleep, nicely tired but not exhausted, it will all help you in your battle against our common enemies of pain and lack of independence. Keep moving and keep your mind occupied as well as managing your diet, for all this will contribute to the new mobile and confident you.

You may say that to be able to get about sufficiently to keep your house clean and attractive and cook appetising meals for your family will be all you ask for. That is fine, as long as you really enjoy doing it and they appreciate you and realise just what an achievement it is for you to return to all that vacuuming, washing, ironing, etc, but I would prefer to see you leave the heavier work to those more able to cope with it and enjoy yourself a little more in some of the ways indicated, even if it is only visiting relatives or neighbours for a chat. In other words, try not to feel guilty about spending some time and effort on yourself as well as enjoying looking after your family, and do not worry about a little chaos in the home.

My approach to helping alleviate the pain of arthritis may seem a trifle simplistic when compared to the major research programmes and orthodox complicated treatments available. *But what is important is that it works.* It has been suggested by some that if you want to get better badly enough and have sufficient faith in the treatment offered, you will get better anyway by means of the placebo effect. If this were true, I feel I would have recovered years ago when desperately trying one so-called cure after another, some orthodox, some fringe-medicine recommended on the grapevine of old wives' tales or word of mouth from others for whom it had been successful. Once the allergic implications of rheumatoid arthritis are recognised, it is easy to see why some treatments succeed in some people and not in others. Although we all have a similar problem, we are all remarkably different and need to be treated individually to suit our own brand of internal chemistry.

Over the years I have been told by people with arthritis or other diseases of quite incorrect advice given to them by their GP or specialist, as well as a lack of simple corrective treatment. Because such interviews are not recorded there is no question of any redress. Naturally, all humans make errors and you cannot expect any doctor to know everything about every medical subject, so it is best if we do not expect too much from them. On general experience it is often difficult to extract many direct answers and one wonders if this professional silence is sometimes designed to cover a lack of knowledge. The best you can do, if worried about your lack of progress, is to obtain as much information as you can from all possible sources and then make your own decisions as to which course to take.

A quite different subject, and one some may feel of secondary importance to one's health, is a visit to the optician. These well appointed premises are in every high street and attended by at least a highly qualified eye specialist, fitter and receptionist. One of my case-histories recently attended for an eye test as he was naturally concerned that occasionally he found it impossible to read and could not focus properly as characters completely disappeared.

After the usual simple tests, he enquired of the visiting specialist the reason for the difficulty he was sometimes experiencing in reading. There was no reply and the patient came away with a prescription for the next strength of lenses for reading but with no reassurance that these could cure the trouble – which was described as merely an intermittent phenomenon.

It may be felt that the majority of the population need to have someone to look up to and respect, such as a prime minister or a boss of some sort, but you should beware of overrating the capabilities of your medical advisor by reading too much into gesture or lack of reply. It all comes back to taking responsibility for your own health and wellbeing and it is part of the positive attitude which helps you to deal directly with any specific illness which has afflicted you. A determined attitude towards your treatment and eventual return to a normal lifestyle will naturally assist in your recovery.

However, I would add that although I tried for many years to keep a cheerful and positive exterior, it was not until I eventually sorted out my diet and became reasonably mentally and physically fit again that my inner confidence and cheerfulness became a reality. I can say with all honesty that, for me at least, arthritis was not all in the mind but in the digestive system.

– 15 –

Losing Weight – And Other Bonuses Of Discovering Your Allergens

I have already discussed the detrimental side effects which can be the result of taking drugs to suppress the various symptoms of rheumatoid arthritis. Now I can take pleasure in enumerating certain fringe benefits which are frequently the result of sorting out your own diet by eliminating those foods which were causing your pain and disability. So far, I have concentrated on rheumatoid arthritis and its alleviation by diet, but other beneficial side effects are well worth a mention. In fact, some people have gone on to a similar diet just to treat these irritating conditions which to people with a serious illness were just something else to be tolerated.

The first bonus which usually arises after allergic people eliminate their allergies, apart from the main one of less pain, is that they start to lose weight. No matter how much they eat of their permitted safe foods, they usually continue to lose weight until they level out at the correct weight for their height and build. It does not seem to make any difference if chips and sweets are eaten, as long as you are not allergic to them.

Just imagine the exhilarating effect this has on your morale, as you lose not only your aches and pains, but all that burdensome fat as well. No wonder there is often a renewed interest in clothes and appearance at the same time! It has been explained to me that this surplus weight is not always fat at all, but mostly retained water. The puffiness of swollen joints is easy to visualise as watery fluid, but apparently what happens in an allergic reaction to the wrong food is that it distends every soft cell in the body with extra fluid. Take away the cause of this enlargement and the fluid gradually flows away, so do not be surprised if you have to pass water more frequently than usual. It is all in a good cause.

It is surprising how many plump people do not over-eat, but simply eat the wrong things for the physical mechanics of their personal make-up. We all know how difficult it is to stop eating our favourite food, be it chocolate, cream cakes, bread and butter, or even bran on our breakfast cereal, sherry, beer, or whatever. However, once you have successfully broken the habits of a lifetime by establishing yourself on a different, but enjoyable diet which alleviates your pain, you will have a very real incentive not to return to your old ways and so your weight should remain at a new low and your morale at a new high. This naturally will be helped by your now being able to take more exercise. For those who are keen enough, special exercises to hold in sagging tummy muscles or bolster the strength and appearance of most other areas can be undertaken.

The Western style of diet is especially bad when it comes to increasing the nation's collective weight. Eastern cultures with their exotic traditions of varied and delicious cuisine do not produce the same problem nor, incidentally, the same incidence of degenerative diseases such as rheumatoid arthritis, heart disease and multiple sclerosis. In trying to analyse the differences between the two main culinary regimes, it appears that in the East food is eaten as fresh as possible, as whole as possible and with the minimum of cooking and maximum variety. A historical shortage of cooking fuel brought about an economical way of cooking food quickly over a bright heat, especially in warmer climates where prolonged cooking heat was unwelcome. In our colder climes the fire was alight all day, so what could be more pleasant than huddling round it baking bread, stirring slow stews and over-cooking vegetables? Traditionally too, the fuels available were slow burning peat or coal, not short-lived twigs and wood.

Climate also plays its part in the crops grown. The more northern climates produce wheat, potatoes, meat and dairy products whilst the warmer areas encourage rice, beans and vegetables. The over-cooking, over-refining and excess processing of foods also play a significant part in the relative health of the consumer, as do the farming methods used. Gardening or smallholding self-supporting communities seem to win in the health stakes every time.

The proportions of starches, vegetables and animal protein eaten are also important, hence my recommendations in Chapter 6 about which foods to eat. When planning and preparing meals, try to avoid over-cooking, enjoy at least one meal a day of raw, fresh salad, a variety of sprouted seeds and shredded vegetables with suitable dressings, very small portions of the meat and fish which you discover will suit you, and plenty of rice, potatoes, beans and nuts which will satisfy your appetite without over-eating. Fruit is sometimes a problem for arthritics but sweet, ripe pears, peaches, bananas, mangoes and grapes are far less likely to upset you than citrus fruit, apples, or soft fruit. You will just have to test carefully each kind in the ways outlined to discover which is safe for you to eat. You may find you can risk certain foods once a week but not every day.

After some years of completely abstaining from certain foods, the allergic reaction to them can in some instances become less severe, enabling you to return to taking just a little of the food or drink as a treat very occasionally. Try it out and note reactions, but do not fall into the trap of thinking you can safely return to eating it all the time or you will find you will experience a replay of long-forgotten aches and pains and have to start all over again with the laborious task of re-breaking addictions. I well remember almost desperately and absurdly clinging to my cups of coffee long after I knew they were making me feel more tired and run-down than was necessary.

Several times I gave coffee up, enjoyed the benefits and then gradually crept back one by one to several cups a day. At last I *think* I have finally got over the longing for it, so I sympathise that your efforts will not be easy.

However, I have successfully tried out the odd bar of chocolate and non-dairy ice cream, plus shop-fried fish and chips, all of which I enjoy as treats now and again with no ill-effects. These are not items to be recommended as healthy, but they are an entrée back into the more humanising world of ordinary food when visiting friends or on excursions where it is necessary to eat in restaurants.

An example of how easy it is to do almost everything towards helping yourself and still not succeed is a lady who consulted me about her arthritis and other troubles. After studying her usual diet, I advised her to first try leaving all dairy products off the menu for a month and report back as to how she was. She duly reported back that she had eaten no cheese, cream, yoghurt, etc, but confessed she had not been able to resist continuing to take milk in her tea. She thought this was an insignificant quantity which would not count. This is a good example of the addictive quality of an allergy, and was unfortunately sufficient to nullify her sterling efforts in other directions because it continued to feed the addiction and prevented her from benefiting. The moral is, it is an all-or-nothing exercise at first, which is the hardest time, although your resolve should be at its strongest. Only after you feel better might it be prudent to relax the regime and try a few experimental treats as outlined.

Fortunately, as already mentioned, there has recently been a lot more interest in the diet we eat. At long last, some publicity is being given to the politics which have actively encouraged the over-consumption of refined sugar and starch and even too much milk, butter and cheese.

Some of your friends and relations, neighbours and well-meaning acquaintances are therefore likely to be full of information about a low fat/sugar diet, rich in fibre and natural nutrients. This will, of course, be helpful in improving the general health of everybody who successfully makes the change, resulting in less weight, more energy and less risk of clogged arteries and heart disease or cancer of the colon. If adopted, ultimately this better eating pattern should also lessen the incidence of people who become allergic to certain over-processed foods which are at present being addictively eaten too frequently. But be careful too of incorrect use of the word 'allergic'. Recently in the press this has been used when a cat refused to drink milk simply because it preferred to drink water. The cat's choice does not mean it was allergic to milk, though it may have had an aversion to it.

But if you are already allergic to certain foods the above change to a generally healthier diet *is not sufficient by itself* for you to feel the very real benefits of tracing the actual items to which your system reacts adversely.

The lists in Chapter 6 are designed to assist you to do this and the 'challenge tests' in Chapter 9 will help you gradually to include other foods which may still suit you. It is only by doing these tests first that people with diseases such as arthritis, eczema and in some cases, multiple sclerosis, can begin to feel better.

Amongst the foods that you can still eat will be some which may be healthier than others, so in these instances you can apply the same general rules as your friends, ie not too many empty calories. This means cutting down on the refined sugar in sweets, cakes, puddings and alcohol, which have had all their goodness in the form of fibre, vitamins and minerals removed. Far better to eat your sugar in its natural form in fruits and vegetables. The same applies to the cereal grains which you discover still suit your particular make-up. Buy unadulterated whole brown flour, rice, corn and so on, which has far more taste and goodness than the white, powdery over-processed and refined types. In other words, do not be misled by a lot of talk about a 'healthy diet', but apply these golden rules to your own individual diet which excludes all the items to which you are allergic.

Tucking in heartily to my new strict regime, thoroughly

enjoying my meals and snacks and never stinting the helpings, I lost enough weight to go down two dress sizes. Seeing the difference more clearly on my visits to them, my parents were concerned I would sink back to the delicacy of the over-thin days early on in my illness, but I felt so well in myself that I had no doubts about the benefits of the loss of weight. After seven years I have increased again by about half a stone, but still take the smaller dress size. The increased weight is mainly in increased muscle quite visible in arms and legs with the benefits very noticeable in my increased ability to lift, bend, clean, unscrew jars and so on. So there you have three main benefits I derived from a change to a managed diet: less pain, less weight and more strength.

Another quite unexpected development and one which makes me suspect rheumatoid arthritis is tied up with women's hormonal make-up was the curious effect on my breasts. For a long time they had been painful, lumpy and had a 'full' feeling with prominent nipples, especially during the week before a period. To my relief, the lumps were diagnosed as not being malignant, but the general condition was termed mastitis; no treatment was available and 'no harm would come to me'. As I said earlier, this was just one more inconvenience to put up with. In retrospect, I should be grateful I had this problem, because it was the 'full' feeling which prompted me to feel I was brimming over with milk and made me suspect that if I stopped drinking it my breasts might feel better. They did. The lumps and pain evaporated along with the joint pains.

While we are on the subject of women's problems, it is frequently found that painful and heavy periods revert to painless, normal happenings with much less pre-menstrual tension when the woman cuts out any foods to which she personally is allergic. I have not taken my previous almost life-long two painkillers a month for some years now, although if I eat anything unwise a day or two before a period I do feel just a little nauseous and off-colour on the first day. Add it up and that is another twelve days a year when you are feeling well instead of decidedly ill, not to mention the bonus of less irritability towards your loved ones before, and the ability to go out with more confidence, after the event.

If you are at all typical, your mental outlook and ability will also change for the better as a result of harmonious dietary control. Forgive me if I keep boasting about how *I* changed, but this is only because it is the best way I can think of to describe this incredible good fortune which has affected every aspect of my life, and to pass on the benefits to others interested. To put it briefly, from being dejected, miserable and depressed, I am now contented, bubbling over with happiness just to be alive and full of enthusiasm for all sorts of projects – some serious, some entirely frivolous. I have become more intensely aware of the beauty around me and the goodness in most other people. From being rather slow in certain types of logic, I can now more quickly understand arguments, follow politics to a certain extent and reason things out which would previously have defeated me. Mathematics never rated very highly in my achievements. Although I still make careless errors, particularly when hurried or flustered, if it is important I can quietly work things out in this area too. I do not give up on problems any more, nor take other people's word for things.

My confidence and self-esteem have also taken a vast turn for the better. All these intangibles are not immediately apparent to an outsider, but to the person concerned they add up to a big improvement in the quality of life. We hear quite a lot in the media nowadays about the treatment of phobias of one sort or another. If you can call an unreasoning fear of darkness, strangers, travel, dogs, etc, a phobia, I have overcome the whole spectrum at a stroke. I now have only a reasonable caution towards all these sorts of things, which can readily be overcome if necessary, even to the extent of tipping up my gumboots before thrusting my foot into them too firmly, since a mouse ran out of one with an equal and opposite speed and direction. I do not know which of us was the more startled; I was just glad he had space to escape before the gap closed entirely!

Back to other fringe advantages. Those previous continuous bruises are not nearly so prominent, nor so frequent, although still occasionally present on only gentle impact. Occasionally, a finger fills up with blood in a rather disconcerting fashion, turning completely black and blue. Often I cannot recall knocking it, although once or twice it has been caused by lifting a bucket with a thin handle, or a parcel by the string. However, it recovers and I usually wear long sleeves and jeans to conceal the rest. Whilst thinking about personal appearance, I would add here that eczema, spots and skin disorders in general usually respond like magic to a prudent diet for arthritis. This is quite contrary to the accepted line given by the establishment specialists in these fields. My own skin is rather dry and I have been fortunate never to have suffered from spots. However, it is rather thin and fragile, but on the whole better than it was. The adverse side effect of steroids, which made my cheeks burn for many years, has abated to bearable proportions, though the damage and broken veins remain and I still flush in an atmosphere which is too warm.

In the main, allergic people seem to have a problem with temperature control. Some always feel too hot, others cannot stand the cold, whilst most dislike either extreme. For years I felt the cold acutely as it seemed to intensify my aches and pains. On the other hand, the longed-for warm summer days drained away the little energy I had, so a happy average was the best to aim for. Nowadays, being more active and in less pain helps to ward off the cold, but I am still distinctly unhappy if the temperature rises too high. I have not been able to find any research in this area and would be interested to hear of other people's reactions to temperature, and their solutions to the problem.

You may have thought I was exaggerating when I said earlier how my dietary approach had affected virtually every aspect of my life and indeed it was not until recently compiling a list for this chapter that I realised how all-pervasive my improvement had been, and in confirmation I have heard from many people similarly placed. It is up to you to see whether similar results come from your treatment of your rheumatoid arthritis.

Who would possibly have imagined that improving my arthritis in this way would affect the health of my teeth? It is not because I clean them more often, though it does occur to me that the mobility and strength of my wrist has improved, so the brushing they get is possibly more effective. It is certainly not through abstaining from sweet sticky things. I enjoy cakes, coconut ice, chocolate, nut toffees, ice cream and so on fairly freely, as long as they have no milk or other forbidden (for me) components in them. Yet from losing quite a few back teeth and having altogether too regular fillings in the rest, nowadays I hardly need to visit the dentist. I hope my bones are strengthening in similar fashion, as one hears such worrying tales of thinning bones in middle-age, together with steroids attacking the bone structure.

The next item on this gleeful list of accidental achievements is hair. Many folk of my age are definitely turning grey. Sister number one will forgive me if I say hers has been that way for some years now, admittedly possibly triggered off by a serious accident injuring one of her children. My hair on the other hand is glossy, healthy and retaining its colour. It used to come out in the hairbrush in the proverbial handful, but it has now thickened up and can be given a good brush through in the morning with hardly a thought for the struggle it used to be. I had a scare recently when it started to shed all over the place again, but when I realised the much advertised medicated shampoo I was using was too strong and reverted back to a purer milder one, it stopped shedding and thickened up again.

A more serious problem I had was with my eyes. We all tend to worry if there is something amiss with our eyes and I am no exception, particularly as I enjoy painting as a hobby and colour and scenery are vital aspects of my life. When my rheumatoid arthritis was very bad I used to comfort myself with the promise that if I eventually became unable to get about at all, I would concentrate on painting. I have no such thoughts now because I am so sure that as long as I keep to my diet I will remain active. Perhaps one day I will have more time to enjoy some painting again, but other things keep me so busy that the prospect seems dim at the moment. It is good to have something like that in hand, though, just in case life should become dull.

Back to the sight problem. I have been blessed with good eyesight throughout my life – in fact at one time I could honestly say my eyes were the only part of me which worked properly; and I have not yet required spectacles even for reading. But after many years of arthritis and steroids they began to get very sore and perpetually bloodshot. Instead of secreting protective tears they dried up and made a lot of sticky gunge which I had to remove and frequently substitute artificial tears from a little bottle. They were also extremely light-sensitive and would smart if I forgot my dark glasses or if a light were switched on suddenly in the night, even if my eyes were tightly closed. Also from time to time I would get a corneal ulcer, which is a lesion in the protective transparent covering of the eye. I felt as if there was something foreign in the eye which would not go away. It was just another worry to add to the main one of rheumatoid arthritis. However, very slowly – so slowly in fact its progress was unnoticed until achieved – the soreness eased, the gunge diminished, the need for artificial tears abated and time between ulcers lengthened. Once again, I hesitate to say I am cured of this particular ill, but I will risk boring you by saying my eyes are so much better I can hardly believe it myself. It is difficult to say which allergen was aggravating my eyes in that way, but I have since read of wheat flour products being implicated in eye disorders in other people.

This list of benefits from dietary control seems to go on and on, but I must just tell you about my stomach ulcer. For years I had indigestion and a gnawing pain and on the doctor's prescription took tablets to calm them, along with frequent snacks of biscuits and milky drinks to keep something in the stomach to neutralise the acids. During 1965, whilst in a London teaching hospital where they were trying to wean me off steroids, I had a barium meal X-ray which confirmed an ulcer. Milk with a beaten egg in it every couple of hours was served along with yet more pills. Needless to say I did not improve and had to cope with the ulcer until about 1976 when during yet another sojourn in hospital another X-ray confirmed it was still there. The staff at this hospital could not understand why I could not tolerate much milk – the then accepted treatment – but salads had no ill-effect. It was very soon after that stay in hospital that I really got down to realising my diet needed drastic revision and the result on the ulcer was virtually instant. I did not need any more X-rays to confirm it had gone.

An interesting side-issue during an early part of my dietary treatment was to ask my doctor to prescribe an antacid tablet without the milk and malt which comprised the bulk of the tablets I had been prescribed for many years and indeed received relief from the stomach pains with. It was a classic case of unwittingly being recommended to take an extra dose of the very irritant which was contributing to the illness in the first place. No wonder doctors are wary of tackling the complex problems of allergy sufferers.

Since the day of my dietary reform, I have had no more ulcer pains. If I get a little indigestion after indiscreet eating, then a piece of raw white cabbage is usually most effective. If none is available, a peppermint antacid tablet, as taken by most of the population at some time, is all that is necessary to restore my inside to its now usual very comfortable state.

Perhaps if you have read this long catalogue of various illnesses so markedly relieved, you may have become sceptical and feel no treatment can be *that* good. But I can only tell you the truth as I see it and leave the conclusions to each individual after giving the therapy a serious trial. I have counted seventeen positive improvements in my life, including the major ones of less pain and more mobility. I have a few restrictions and problems left which I am still working on, but from being a grumpy, pain-racked misery I am now cheerful, almost free of pain and full of optimism for the future. Consequently, for me it is well worth limiting some of the variety of foods I once ate. I have never counted my blessings quite so exactly until now – when even I am surprised at the variety and number of them.

It just depends on how ill you are and how desperate to recover as to whether or not you persevere with what could possibly be a rather anti-social diet. It need not be too limiting if you tackle it positively, seek adequate alternatives and interest friends and relatives in your aims so they know what to serve you on visits. At least you know all the possibilities now and can make a choice between pain and indulgence.

– 16 –

How Things Are Now

I frequently awaken at 6 am and just occasionally am tempted to go out when I find it is one of those lovely early spring mornings with the mist lying over the fields and remnants of frost being burnt off by a red ball of sun rising over the river. Who could go back to the temptations of a warm bed on such a day? Quickly donning jeans and a jersey, I slip silently out of the house before I am missed.

The air is as fresh as champagne. No other human sound spoils the moment. As quietly as possible, so as not to break the spell, I unlock the shed to get oars, rowlocks and buoyancy aid. Moving the dinghy and shipping the oars and rowlocks magnifies bumps and noises which seem too loud to escape the notice of sleepers within, but I carefully kneel and lower my weight into the centre of the little craft and we are away. By this time there is warmth and brightness in the sun reflecting back off the ripples made on the calm water. I am overjoyed to be afloat again after a long, dull winter.

We drift aimlessly on the current for a while absorbing the silence of the moment, then grasping the oars I lean forward, dip the blades in and pull with all my strength, combining weight with the muscle power I used not to have. The light craft shoots forward in immediate response. Again and again I pull on the oars, terminating each stroke with a jerk to extract all the speed of which we are capable. We plough rhythmically through the water with that unique rippling, rushing sound until my mouth goes dry with the exertion and the time has come to rest. We drift into the side, now out of sight of any habitation and my exhilaration calms to a quiet appreciation of the scene. I am content to gaze and gaze.

A reed bunting, tame and inquisitive, is busy amongst the dry, straw-like winter reeds. Skylarks sing high overhead in the sunshine. After a while a bank vole cautiously pops his head out of his hideaway I hold my breath. Reassured, he gets on with his daily business of cutting the 'lawn' around the burrow and taking breakfast below in little bundles. The chances are there is a young family down there and, although tiny, these creatures eat an endless supply of fresh green vegetable matter, chickweed being the favourite.

A gentle breeze is getting up with the sun and it catches the dinghy, turning it away from the bank. It and the current take us round the next bend. Endless miniature vistas unfold, familiar and much visited places rendered fresh and new in the early morning light.

As the sun gets stronger, so the special moment fades. Reluctantly, I row my boat towards home, tie her up and return to dry land. The postman cycles past and without stopping puts the bundle of letters into my outstretched hand.

There were many years when I could not get into a tippy dinghy, even with helpers to steady the boat for me. At one time I even had difficulty just stepping aboard a much larger, more stable craft.

Naturally, most of my days begin here. I wake with no morning stiffness or pain, refreshed after the night's rest (unless I overstrained some joint the previous day, or ate the wrong food). I do not sleep continuously through the night, but am rarely bothered about lying awake for an hour or so. I let my mind roam over past and planned events, while continuing to doze and rest. It used to take at least two hours for me to wash, dress, breakfast and be ready for the then restricted events of the day, and that was really working hard at it and finishing exhausted and in need of a sit-down. Nowadays it takes an hour at most, without hurrying at all.

Washing is a joy because I can reach all round my neck with my left hand, and even the right arm, in which the joints still do not work sufficiently to be so mobile, has the strength to give its opposite number a good rub. I can still reach my feet to attend to them and get in and out of the bath unassisted. What is more, I can stoop to reach and clean it afterwards.

I used to have to bend over and gradually pull nighties, jumpers, and other clothes over my head in a painfully frustrating way. Now, if they are light and loose enough, I can stand upright and lift them up and over in a near normal action. As I said, washing, brushing and attending to my hair are no longer problems, but pleasures.

It is difficult to choose a typical day because my activities vary so much. Some days I can do relatively much more, but then need a relaxed day to recover. I nearly always answer a few letters straight onto the typewriter, or type out an article or a chapter. I enjoy doing this as I love to communicate. I cannot cope if there is too much continuous typing to be done, because any activity carried out too long tends to make the joints and muscles which are being used over-tired and painful. In this case especially, arms, neck and back ache from the tensing of the muscles to maintain position and concentration.

If the weather is at all inviting I look around for a more active outdoor task: perhaps cutting the grass with an electric mower, a little digging or weeding or painting. Repairing concrete paths, refelting or replacing tiles on roofs also come into my repertoire now, but again though I enjoy the challenge and satisfaction of these pursuits, I can only do a little at a time and often pay for my pleasures with increased aches and pains, together with bruises from clambering across ladders on hands and knees. Overall, I feel these little adventures increase my fitness and general well-being and are much better than under-utilising joints and energy.

You may have noticed housework comes low on my list of priorities. Naturally I do this too, but do not allow a wish for cleanliness and order to absorb all my time and energy.

Housework seems rather an unrewarding task as the rooms soon look dusty and untidy again. Vacuum cleaning still soon exhausts me and gives me backache, as do ironing or window cleaning. However, by doing a job in short bursts a tolerable compromise can be reached. It is a case of rationing out available energy for the most benefit in satisfaction to yourself and family, together with progress in any other tasks you wish to undertake.

At the risk of sounding as if I am complaining, I have noticed that it is frequently the people who need them most who do not have all the latest gadgets to take the hard work out of living. A washing machine and food processor, for instance, would save your strength for more pleasurable things whilst keeping your standards high – if not bringing them higher than you were able to manage before. Sink and worktop heights, cupboards and floors can all be tailor-made for comfort, besides ease of cleaning. A woman to come in and do some of the more heavy household chores just once a week should not be beyond most budgets, or if it really is, have you asked your doctor if you qualify for a home-help? Failing either of these approaches, are the rest of the household as helpful as they might be in saving you doing repetitive and wearying tasks?

Do put your own needs high on your list of priorities. I know it is not easy to change your ways in this respect. For instance, if I were suggesting you cooked a special diet for your husband or child, or saved them from tiring chores, you would probably agree with enthusiasm if you felt it would help make them feel better. However, because it is for yourself, you are probably wondering if you can spare the time and effort, especially if it means a little less attention to the comfort of others. But you are important too; your own health is vital for your family and they will benefit eventually and appreciate having you feeling better.

From being quiet, introverted, depressed and grumpy, I have become more outgoing and confident, laugh a lot and am full of ideas and enthusiasm for various projects and outings. I know my personality and habits have changed over the last few years, but I am the first to agree the change has not been for the better in all respects. At one time I loved to cook our family's favourite meals for us to enjoy together. Now I look at the rich ingredients which made me so ill and cannot bring myself to serve them for family or guests very often. Worse, from their point of view, if I am too busy to do all the baking, my bread and cakes often come first and others have to make do with shop wholemeal bread and more simple, quicker meals (but not convenience foods full of additives). I used to be an agreeable person to live with because I had hardly any strong opinions of my own and would allow myself, because it was easier, to be carried along by others. Suddenly I find this is not good enough and will defend my point of view to the surprise and chagrin of those close to me. My time has also become more valuable and I have had to insist on the time to write and gradually type this book, or answer letters from correspondents with arthritis and so on. This does not always make for peace and harmony, but you are a person in your own right and deserve better treatment than a much-loved doormat. The time has come to take the course of your life into your own hands and improve your health through your own efforts with or without the active co-operation of others close to you. You can do it. Just work out all the ways and means and announce that this is what you are going to do and press on regardless of any outcry or derision. Try to keep a calm and cheerful outlook, sympathise with them a little, but do not be deflected from your purpose. Once others realise you are indeed serious and they can see your health improve, they will come round to your way of thinking.

Although I would not, of course, have volunteered to undergo the illness I have had, I do believe the experiences have made me far more tolerant and understanding of others and have shaped my character so that I am a different person to the one I would have been had I led an entirely healthy and uneventful life.

So – consider your own needs a little more and the needs of others a little less. It will repay you in the long run and help you to feel better and to put some of your new-found energy into your own more absorbing hobbies, or into sharing a pleasurable day out with the family at a more active level. Friends and family will eagerly welcome you as an active and cheerful participant once more. However much good friends, workmates and family sympathise with your misfortunes, they cannot fully understand and have to continue in their more active life, thus tending to grow away from you. Your relationship is damaged right from the start if you dare not shake hands on meeting for fear of the pain and cannot undertake a cuddle or a little horseplay for similar reasons. Physical withdrawal of this sort gives the impression you do not wish to be friendly, and that you do not care for the person or child concerned. It is not always possible to put all your real feelings of love or friendship into words they will understand. What I am really saying is that only you know how ill and incapacitated you are and it is up to *you* to obtain as much actual assistance as possible, be it mechanical or human, to release you to enjoy life again.

I used to be a worrier, I must admit, but now I feel so much better in all other aspects, due entirely to my changed diet, that I find I hardly worry at all. Everything has fallen into a new perspective and any worrying I do is of a more constructive nature. I do, of course, have a full share of trials and tribulations quite unconnected with my health. Such events used to quite set me back. Now, even when my home is threatened with demolition by planning authorities, I simply fight back and even relish the fight, although it has taken up an undue share of my precious ration of active time and energy.

You may hear that rheumatoid arthritis can be triggered off or made worse by stress. But in my own experience any anxiety present seems to be a part of and heightened by the disease, rather than the outside stress aggravating it. Part of the allergy syndrome is connected with the mind and moods of the victim, in addition to the more visible symptoms of swelling and deformity.

Back to a typical day. After a lunch, usually mainly of salad and raw vegetables as available in the different seasons, I try – and usually succeed – to resist the delicious sleepy feeling that creeps over me and go shopping or visiting. I learned to drive as soon as I was old enough, thanks to my father's perseverance, but alas for many years was only a passenger and could not raise my hands far enough even to clear the windscreen of mist for the benefit of the driver. I simply had neither the strength nor confidence even to think of driving. Quite soon after I eliminated all dairy products from my diet, I was well enough physically to want to drive, and as we only had a Land Rover at the time, I was thrown in at the deep end. I eventually got used to short trips in quiet lanes and was delighted to be able to go shopping or post a letter independently again. The joy of bowling along in such a bumpy vehicle was only equalled by being able to see over hedges never seen over before and by the looks on men's faces as I parked perilously near their precious shiny cars.

The increased traffic since I last drove and the speed of manoeuvring and tight parking in towns is quite another thing and I am still getting used to these, even though I now have a small saloon. Also, once again I can only drive for a short while at a time and a round trip of 25 miles with errands at the other end leaves me feeling rather limp. It is partly the physical effort involved, partly the nervous energy, but well worth the exertion for the feeling of independence and self-esteem engendered.

In order really to appreciate these simple pleasures of everyday living, it is first necessary to be deprived of them. Rather like a person who has been stranded in the desert or at sea with nothing to drink, you never again take for granted the simple things like a drink of water. It is impossible to really savour the highlights of life without first experiencing something of the low spots. Although I would naturally rather not have been ill for so long, the despair which I endured has taught me many things, including tolerance and to live each day with as much pleasure as possible. I do not mean one should live in a selfish or expensive way, but that sharing happiness with others in very simple ways, such as a pleasant exchange of words in a shop, a job well done, or a chat with an elderly neighbour, brings immense joy and satisfaction.

Maybe I am a bit old fashioned, but I think the same sort of principles apply to the acquiring of possessions or taking holidays abroad. School children are nowadays taken on all sorts of wonderful trips and given many sporting opportunities. Their parents, or rate and tax payers, work hard to pay for these and often never have the same opportunities themselves. I wonder if the youngsters fully appreciate their privileged position or whether they simply grow up expecting more and more treats without the need to work and save first. To have some aim in life to work towards seems a desirable part of the human make-up, be it a career, a special hobby like mountaineering or sailing, marriage and gradually building up a new home and children, or just the desire to travel abroad. If all these things are provided too easily while still young, what is there left to strive for and look forward to?

For example, I have been lucky to go out with many first-time sailors and it is a pleasure to see the enjoyment and satisfaction derived by some of the older ones, who at their own expense are realising a life-time's ambition before my eyes. This can be compared to the blasé, even lazy attitude of some who think they will just try the sport in passing, amongst their many other diversions.

In the depth of winter I will find an excuse to go out every day, even if only for a short while. With frost and snow on the ground everywhere looking so lovely I revert to a childhood pleasure of treading footprints into virgin snow. Naturally I feed the birds. Our waterbirds tend to have different needs to those on the usual bird table, but the bluetits and great-tits find their way to the rather isolated offerings of fat and nuts. They reward me by nesting in little boxes specially built into the walls of the house. I often watch their antics and wonder if all that suet is damaging their tiny hearts. But as soon as spring comes they lose interest in dead food and provide their fledglings with hundreds of green caterpillars. I search the garden yet cannot find any. They must have exceptional eyesight.

When the water freezes over, wading and swimming birds are in great distress. Even if a small area stays open for the divers, the shyer, rarer birds will not come over for scraps, and these are quickly devoured by the resident ducks and swooping seagulls. In periods of deep frosts more and more little corpses lie on the ice which is often too thick to get a boat through and too thin to trust to walk upon, so there was no way to reach a pair of swans which rested on the ice one night and became frozen to it by morning. Fortunately, it was a bright sunny day and they eventually struggled free to come over for some bread and water where I could reach to break the ice for them.

The question of suitable food for semi-tame waterbirds of this sort weighs heavily when raising the various orphans and injured birds which come my way. Contributions are received of enriched baby food and fish fingers for starving birds. Supposedly eaters of waterweeds and fish they spurn offerings of the food which is supposed to be good for them and, like their human counterparts, gobble up cornflakes and bread together with petshop pellets of wheat.

Given a bowl of tap water most day-old ducklings refuse to swim, but one orphan, soon after hatching, was given a bowl with some waterweed in it. He dived in and filtered out all the shrimp which had been clinging to the weed in a most efficient manner, then preened himself dry for hours afterwards. He had never seen shrimps before, nor other ducks preening, but he grew up with all the skills and attributes of his breed, even eventually bringing a little 'wife' along each day to share his food.

At the end of an ordinary-sounding day, by the time I have prepared and eaten the evening meal, I am usually too tired to do much else but read or watch television. After a rest I gather the strength to wash the dishes of the entire day. When I was too weary to wash up as I went along I used to do it all in the morning in very hot water to try to ease my stiff fingers and wrists. As that exercise is now unnecessary, in the mornings I put the hygienically rinsed and air-dried dishes away while I am waiting for the toast and start my day that much earlier than I used to.

I still seem to need a longer night's rest than most people, so often go to bed before 10 pm usually nicely tired, but not in pain. Before dropping off to sleep I relive the events of the day and work out schemes for achieving more of my remaining ambitions, which should have been worked through while young.

Most of all, I give thanks for my deliverance from pain.

Conclusion

My main ambition is to see an increasing number of people with arthritis, particularly the young ones, derive as much benefit and relief as I have done from the simple and safe measures described in this book. So here they are again, the seven steps to happiness:

1. Your first step, and the most important one for arthritics, is to try an initial period strictly on the elimination diet especially evolved for people with arthritis as described in Chapter 6.
2. Clean up your chemical environment at home and at work by providing an oasis relatively free of pollution. Banish all aerosols, highly perfumed products, strong chemical cleaners, smokers.
3. Stop taking painkilling tablets as soon as they become unnecessary, and consult your medical advisor to assist you to reduce other medications if your improvement persists.
4. Take more exercise and positive action to enjoy yourself and extend your capabilities as described in Chapter 14.
5. Challenge your new-found state of health with the foods you have not been eating, testing each item strictly one by one until you know for certain which ones you are allergic to.
6. Live and eat in a generally more healthy way, as reiterated throughout.
7. Tell your friends of your good fortune and how you

regained your health. Write to us to help our statistics become recognised in order to help others avoid the unnecessary pain and frustration of this disease.

Useful Addresses

Action Against Allergy
Secretary: Mrs Aeronwy Thomas Ellis, 43 The Downs, London SW20 8HG
Promotes the study of the causative role of foods and chemicals in chronic illness.

Chemical Victims
Secretary: Mrs Shirley Hedges, 12 Highlands Road, Worting, Basingstoke, Hants.
A club for sufferers from food and chemical allergy and for the promotion of the study of clinical ecology in Britain.

Environmental Therapy Research
Standard Chartered Bank Building, 28 Northumberland Avenue, London WC2N 5AG
Advises and exchanges information about allergic reactions and treatments.

Help Yourself to Less Pain Society
Patricia Byrivers, Help Yourself to Less Pain Society, c/o 16 Poynter Road, Bush Hill Park, Enfield, Middlesex EN1 1DN.
Specialises in natural holistic health treatment for allergic arthritis and environmentally or nutritionally induced illness.

Society for Environmental Therapy
Secretary: A. Beckingham, 31 Sarah St, Darwen, Lancashire.
Aims to discover environmental causes of disease and encourage communication between professional and lay public.

Bibliography

Other books which may help you to understand and trace your allergies:

Chemical Victims Dr Richard Mackarness (Pan, 1980)
Not All In The Mind Dr Richard Mackarness (Pan, 1978)
5 Day Allergy Relief System Dr M. Mandell and Lynn Scanlon (Arrow, 1983)
Help Yourself to Less Pain Erick James and Patricia Byrivers (Help Yourself to Less Pain Society, 1983)

Cookery books containing useful recipes which can be adapted for a restricted diet:

The Coeliac Handbook The Coeliac Society
Deliciously Low Harriet Roth (Century, 1984)
Good Food: Grain-free, Milk-free Hilda Cherry Hills (Roberts, 1977)
Indian Cooking Savitri Chowdhary (Andre Deutsch, 1954; Pan 1975) or any other good Indian cookery books
Vegetarian Dishes from the Middle East Arto der Haroutunian (Century, 1983)
virtually any good Chinese cookbook